*Under the Rattlesnake*

CONTEMPORARY AMERICAN INDIAN STUDIES
Heidi M. Altman, *Series Editor*
J. Anthony Paredes, *Founding Editor*

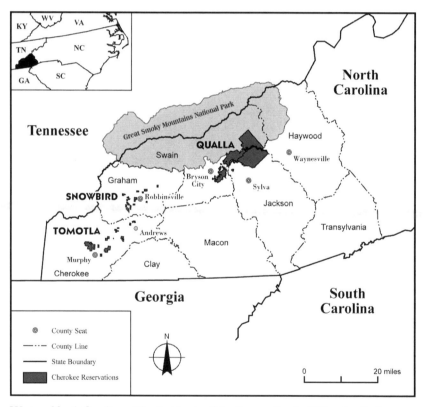

Western North Carolina with tribal lands of the Eastern Band of Cherokee Indians.

# Under the Rattlesnake

## Cherokee Health and Resiliency

Edited by
Lisa J. Lefler

Foreword by
Susan Leading Fox
(Eastern Band of Cherokee Indians)

THE UNIVERSITY OF ALABAMA PRESS

*Tuscaloosa*

Copyright © 2009
The University of Alabama Press
Tuscaloosa, Alabama 35487-0380
All rights reserved
Manufactured in the United States of America

Typeface: ACaslon

∞

The paper on which this book is printed meets the minimum requirements of
American National Standard for Information Sciences-Permanence of Paper for
Printed Library Materials, ANSI Z39.48-1984.

Library of Congress Cataloging-in-Publication Data

Under the rattlesnake : Cherokee health and resiliency / edited by Lisa J. Lefler ;
foreword by Susan Leading Fox (Eastern Band of Cherokee Indians).
    p.   cm. — (Contemporary American Indian studies)
  Includes bibliographical references and index.
    ISBN 978-0-8173-1649-5 (cloth : alk. paper) — ISBN 978-0-8173-5529-6 (pbk. :
alk. paper) — ISBN 978-0-8173-8158-5 (electronic) 1. Indians of North America—
Health and hygiene. 2. Cherokee Indians—Medicine. I. Lefler, Lisa J.
  RA448.5.I5U523 2009
  610.89′97557—dc22

                                                                    2008043152

For my father, Buddy (1930–2006), and my mother, Jean, and all mountain people who have left us with a colorful and rich heritage.

# Contents

# Illustrations

Figures

Tables

# Foreword

*Susan Leading Fox, EBCI Deputy Health Officer*

Shiyo! (Hello!)

An opportunity has been afforded me to share my voice about this book on Cherokee health. And while it is not so unique today, during the time period in which I was born it was not common at all for someone who was Cherokee and white to be asked her opinion about such an important issue. My background and culture is of mixed heritage: Cherokee and Appalachian. While both have their specific experiences and often share values and beliefs, for this purpose I focus on my native heritage. Both cultures depended on God's gifts to provide them with the tools necessary for healing. However, it was up to individuals to map out how or whether they would use the tools taught in our culture. Most information regarding healing was passed down by word of mouth or by teaching useful everyday practices. Unfortunately, today the majority of this information is anecdotal and has been melded into a combination of Native, Appalachian, and Western medicine.

Regardless of what new information is currently available, a foundational principle of Cherokee culture remains: healing cannot occur without an intrinsic connection to something larger than the individual. However, this spiritual connection was not something that occurred on a scheduled day of the week with specific documented rituals, only to be put away until the next appointment; instead we recognized that "connectedness" with all things was a constant. We embraced an individualized relationship with the Creator and with all living things in existence, and understood our responsibilities in those relationships and how our behaviors and intentions could affect our well-being physically and emotionally as well as others around us. Both native people and Appalachian people knew that all living things had a place of value in the circle of life. How this innate awareness of our surroundings and our relationship with this place came to be for our people is unknown, but we believe it was given freely by the very Creator who also provided the means to maintain wellness.

Regardless of how it came about, our knowledge of the gifts the plants and animals provided us was based on a connection to a larger force and relied on awareness of our place in that system of life and death. Maintaining a close, spiritual relationship with the environment and surroundings allowed us to see beauty, usefulness, and gifts in all of creation. The realization that creation was for us to use assumes an enormous responsibility as caretakers of the gifts that were given. If we fail to nurture the world we were gifted, then the system will crumble and fail us all. If you honor that belief, then you too are horrified by the large-scale destruction that is now occurring across the world in the form of human-instigated "natural" disasters and the slow but sure demise of entire ecosystems.

However, the value system that does not recognize our responsibility to the place we occupy has been evident for over five hundred years. When Contact occurred, this system was broken and knowledge that should have been passed on was lost or misinterpreted as a result of families being torn apart, the death of knowledge keepers, and a basic change of lifestyle from living in harmony and honor with one's surroundings to one of dominance for survival.

With that said, Cherokee people have historically been open and welcoming to outsiders, both native and non-native. They acknowledged and appreciated the introduction of new tools, information, and systems that made life easier and richer. It is only when the practices and policies of governments interfered with those networks that relationships became strained and Cherokee people could not afford to be as trusting. As a result of events that occurred outside the control of the Cherokee, an entire set of principles and practices was destroyed. Much of the healing arts was lost or forgotten, causing the connection to creation and the vital spiritual thread that is woven throughout creation to be severely damaged.

Health was defined by standards determined by the federal government along with prescribed cures with little or no confidence placed in cultural medicines or remedies. Paradoxically, new pharmacopeias were provided to Europeans from the wealth of medicinal plants exported after Contact (i.e., ginseng, sassafras, and witch hazel). While these "solutions" and treaty-supported health care provided via federal policy were not entirely harmful in and of themselves, what resulted was a deep dependency on government ideals and services at the expense of the Cherokee's relationship to the spiritual world and its connection to health and wellness.

It is refreshing to see a compilation as is provided here that not only recognizes the existence of Cherokee health and healing but supports its importance in the system of wellness. The discussions of how we perceive the notions of health, wellness, and disease; how we rely on our language to teach us what our elders knew about these relationships; how we deal with the end of the life cycle; and how we are mobilizing both health professionals and community members to deal with contemporary health issues are important for all of us. I encourage you to discover this unique and beautiful relationship of humans to nature through a spiritual connection that will ultimately result in wellness—not only for humans but all of our relations, and, more important, for the very physical world on which our health depends.

Sgi! (Thank you!)

*Under the Rattlesnake*

# Introduction

*Lisa J. Lefler*

> There was an order to things . . . they happened in a way they were sup-
> posed to. There's a natural process of life and we strive to keep our world
> in balance. When we act out of balance, the elders say "human beings
> don't do that." Elders say you can do anything too much. Anything ob-
> sessive takes you away from reality and taking away from reality is im-
> balance.
> —Mr. Tom Belt, Oklahoma Cherokee

Because I am fortunate to have an Appalachian heritage, most of the lessons
that have guided the important things in my life have come from an understanding that we have a relationship with our surroundings: mountains, rivers, and the wide diversity of flora and fauna of the region. My mother is
a mountain woman who knows the sacredness of place and gifts that the
mountains and their ecosystems have to offer. Her knowledge of local plants
was an invaluable resource for a family that had little access to "Western"
medical care. She also understands the spiritual nature of mountains, rivers,
and streams, and always finds solace in them. Her gift to me was an appre-
ciation and knowledge of these resources.

Sharing knowledge, experience, and culture is something that has taken
place in western North Carolina since Contact. But today more than ever,
those of us who have the privilege of knowing and working with people
of the Eastern Band of Cherokee Indians (EBCI) realize we are guests of
this region. We are honored by the friendships, which many Appalachian
people have had with the Cherokees, and value their hospitality and knowledge gained by living here for thousands of years. Our work together on this
book demonstrates this unique relationship; the title, *Under the Rattlesnake,*
was given by one of the Cherokee contributors, Tom Belt. I asked him what
came to mind when he thought about Cherokee health, and he said that
"the rattlesnake was one of the Cherokee's great medicinal symbols. It has
an omnipresence in Cherokee culture, with many meanings: great health, as
well as death. Rattlesnake medicine was very strong and only a few knew

how to administer it. It was taboo to wear its skin. If you did, you could be struck by lightning. The diamond figures on its back are not considered diamond shapes but two concentric lightning strikes. The other significance is that Cherokee proper is located just under Rattlesnake Mountain."

This volume is a direct result of this reciprocal friendship and any proceeds that come as a result of its publication will be forwarded to the EBCI Diabetes Clinic on the Qualla Boundary. I am particularly grateful to Susan Leading Fox, deputy health officer for the EBCI, Renissa Walker, director of the EBCI Kituwah Preservation and Education Program, and T. J. Holland, director and curator for the Junaluska Museum in Robbinsville. Without their assistance, this volume would not have been possible. I would also like to thank two mentors who have provided me with invaluable advice and guidance. Dr. Tony Paredes and Dr. Ray Fogelson are two icons in this field and have unselfishly shared their expertise and good old common sense.

Having experienced the power that plants have to offer, the power of history to guide, and the power that sharing beliefs can heal, the contributors to this volume exemplify these ideals and together have contributed, through this volume, to the fields of anthropology and Cherokee studies. The intent of this book is to provide a true "four-field" approach to understanding health and disease.

Anthropology, referred to as the "holistic" social science, undertakes the huge task of studying the totality of the human experience by breaking the discipline down into four subfields: linguistics, physical or biological anthropology, archaeology, and sociocultural anthropology. These fields overlap, but scholars in each bring four different lenses with which we examine and contemplate issues. An example of how this works is exemplified through this volume, which we hope provides insight into the complicated and connected nature of health among one population, the Eastern Band of Cherokee Indians. Anthropologists, both Native and non-Native, bring their expertise to examine issues of Cherokee health from a variety of perspectives with an array of skills and experiences. Native contributors are able to provide insight that only Natives can, which is essential for any text of this genre. The rest of us are grateful for the privilege of working with Cherokee people and appreciate our collaborative opportunities and friendships. Other contributors in this volume who are not anthropologists provide the interdisciplinary expertise that broadens the field of Cherokee studies.

The incentive for bringing these essays together was an organized panel for the annual meeting of the Appalachian Studies Association, held in Cherokee, North Carolina, in 2004. The conference theme, "Building a

Healthy Region: From Historical Trauma to Hope and Healing," seemed appropriate for a series of papers discussing the health of the Eastern Cherokees since about 1500 A.D., referred to simply as Contact. Our panel discussant, Dr. Raymond D. Fogelson, initially began his fieldwork in Cherokee in the late 1950s and has provided insight and comments on the essays collected here. Dr. Fogelson's work includes topics from Cherokee conjuring to politics to ball play, which has influenced the development of Cherokee studies for more than a half century. His observations and guidance are reflected in these pages and we are grateful for his participation.

The conference keynote speaker was Native psychologist Dr. Eduardo Duran, a friend and "relative," as he refers to himself in the "Indian way." His message concerned the impact of intergenerational trauma and the importance of how to address issues of disease, social pathologies, and mental health through a "de-colonizing" paradigm. His recent text, *Healing the Soul Wound* (2006), is an extension of his presentation and is exemplary of a much-needed paradigm shift in counseling methodology, particularly with Native peoples, but applies to most of us as well. His talk, historically targeting American Indian audiences, was well received by Appalachian scholars and most were introduced that day to a new way of thinking about our overall health and wellness.

The conference taught me something else: to be more careful about what I "think" I know and to be aware of the consequences of having only a "little knowledge." As panel organizer, I was responsible for making all panelists aware of tribal protocol, particularly when referring to human remains. After the papers were read, it was brought to our attention that the room in which we were presenting, which was located in the local high school, would have to be smudged or cleansed before classes could resume the next morning. I was embarrassed and felt I had let my distinguished colleagues down. I knew there would probably be some slides of skeletal remains shown in the discussion of health and/or presence of disease among the early inhabitants of Cherokee territory, but I didn't think that would violate any current tribal protocol. I was wrong.

Unfortunately my colleagues had to bear the brunt of my unfamiliarity regarding discussion of human remains, even though we were in an academic setting. As a result, two of the chapters in this volume include the discussion that should preclude that uncomfortable position in the future. Michelle D. Hamilton and Russell G. Townsend, both of whom were EBCI Tribal Historic Preservation Officers (THPO) at the time, have contributed very important chapters (one chapter by both authors, one by Hamilton) that have been a long time coming for many of us who are interested in studying the human condition of Cherokee peoples at and after Contact. These two chapters expand and update the discussions of Raymond D. Fogelson's articles "An Analysis of Cherokee Sorcery and Witchcraft" (1975) and "Change, Persistence, and Accommodation in Cherokee Medico-Magical Beliefs" (1961), John Witthoft's "Cherokee Beliefs Concerning Death" (1983), and Brett Riggs's "In the Service of Native Interests: Archaeology for, of, and by Cherokee People" (2002).

I am also reminded of the foundational work of Harriet Kupferer (1966), who included issues of contemporary health in her work during the 1950s, which culminated in the classic, *The "Principal People," 1960: A Study of Cultural and Social Groups of the Eastern Cherokee.* Kupferer provides a foundation for other medical anthropologists in the field with her nuanced descriptions and attention to intertribal differences. She represents traditional ethnographic research at its best and set a high standard for those who would follow.

Challenged with more and more projects that require removal of land surface and change in landscape in and around Cherokee historic sites, the EBCI THPO is well aware of the two-edged sword of "development." The largest excavation in the state of North Carolina was being conducted at the Ravensford site on the Qualla Boundary as this volume was in process. Now completed, an executive summary of the excavation, "The Ravensford Tract Archeological Project," by Bennie Keel (2007) represents the progressive collaborative efforts of tribal, state, and federal agencies working together to interpret and preserve Cherokee history. In the process, archaeologists and others involved in like projects must be intimately cognizant of not only the protocol in working on sites with human remains, but also how Cherokees must feel and react to what is being done. The dead must be honored as we strive to learn as much as we can about the history, legacy, and resiliency of the Cherokee people. Hamilton and Townsend contribute information providing an essential context, which must be understood preceding any work that might incur human remains.

Health and diet are, of course, inextricably linked. Not since Mary Story's dissertation (1980), which includes diet inventories, or food frequency questionnaires of Snowbird Cherokees has there been any analysis of diet and disease among the Eastern Band. Ethnobotanist David N. Cozzo provides an overview of many of the traditional foods used by the Cherokees and the nutritional value they possess in combating current health problems. He wisely does not suggest a complete turn back to the sixteenth century.

However, he does suggest serious inquiry into the cultivation and harvesting of some food sources that could be beneficial today. The Eastern Band has a proven history of adaptability and forward thinking in dealing with a rapidly changing world, and their response in dealing with endemic health problems such as diabetes is no different. Their diabetes clinic and prevention program employs nutritionists and paradigms that welcome a fusion of old and new foods. Diabetes patients can also take advantage of complimentary strategies such as acupuncture, message therapy, and yoga. Their bottom line is eat in moderation, get plenty of exercise, and try to reduce stress.

Heidi M. Altman, a linguistic anthropologist, and Thomas N. Belt, Cherokee language coordinator and instructor at Western Carolina University, work together in their chapter to examine the use of Cherokee language in historical and contemporary contexts that describe the relationship of people to the environment. Change and modernity has impacted the availability of resources, inhibited the use of language among the Cherokees (until recent revitalization efforts), and reduced the number of people who write and apprentice with sacred texts. Altman and Belt survey words, terms, and concepts that are part of the unique Cherokee perspective regarding health and wellness and share critical views that represent traditional worldviews of interconnectedness and holism.

More specifically, in this chapter they propose that the contemporary concept of *tōhi:* ("well-being" in Cherokee) is crucial to understanding the ethnohistorical record of interactions between the Cherokee people and European diseases. The chapter explores linguistic examples of the *tōhi:* concept, its relationship to worldview and healing practices, and the light it sheds on historical accounts of Cherokee medicine. In English notions of wellness pertain almost exclusively to either the physical or psychological health of an individual. In some cases this concept is extended to include what some call "quality of life issues" such as the sustainability of a particular standard of living, but in general terms to inquire about a person's wellness is to ask how they are feeling. We most often interpret "well" as simply the adverbial form of "good."

In North Carolina Cherokee, the common greeting is "Siyo! Tōhi-tsu?" or "Hello, are you well?" On the surface this appears to parallel the English "Hello, how are you?" and in fact, the greeting is often glossed this way. However, if one looks more deeply at the concepts encompassed by the word *tōhi* it becomes apparent that *tōhi* is an approximation of the traditional Cherokee view of the workings of the cosmos and the position of the individual in relationship to the rest of the world.

As a medical anthropologist I have been privileged to work on the Qualla Boundary off and on since 1989. For almost five years I worked with a diabetes prevention program funded by the Centers for Disease Control and Prevention and was awed by the resiliency and vision of those in Cherokee who are fighting the battle of diabetes. These contemporary warriors support each other, walk and exercise with each other, and cajole each other every day to watch what they eat and drink and be a role model to their children and grandchildren. The EBCI have learned that diabetes can be controlled and prevented, but many have also learned that how they deal with daily stress and intergenerational trauma can have as much impact as exercising and watching their diet. The chapter I cowrote with Roseanna Belt looks at a grassroots wellness movement whose message of historic and intergenerational trauma has impacted not only their community but many of their health providers and others around them. With a significant diabetes prevalence rate, the EBCI are concerned about their future, including the future of their children and the rising health care costs that increase each year as younger and younger children are diagnosed with Type 2 diabetes. Keeping the model of intergenerational trauma in mind when addressing public health issues, a more holistic approach to prevention and intervention methodologies can be more culturally appropriate when providers understand the impact of colonization and assimilation on health. Paradoxically, remembering the past allows these communities to plan and strategize how to deal with health and social issues. As we learn more about disease causality and prevention we cannot underestimate the importance of the intersection of environment and biology.

Jenny James, a religious studies scholar, looks at the importance of the sacred feminine among traditional Cherokee and traces the use of myth and symbolism to revisit questions regarding the prominence of the feminine within this strong matrilineal culture. Using an interdisciplinary hermeneutical methodology drawn from the history of religions, contextual theology, ethnoastronomy, ecofeminism, and depth psychology, James describes the comprehensive manner in which Cherokee mythology and religion is matriarchal in psychological orientation, matrifocal in cultural meaning, and matrilineal in social power. As many in the community have noted, true healing and progressive change will not happen without the support and contributions of Cherokee women. For young Cherokee women, finding the strength of a matrifocal worldview is essential in building positive self-esteem and self-worth, which guides positive life choices.

By examining standard texts long known to scholars with an interdisciplinary apparatus informed by the sacred woman and dog moiety, James has shown significant religious links between Cherokee culture and the cultures of other Eastern Woodland tribes. In the present essay, she uses one formula from the Swimmer Manuscript to outline the manner in which Cherokee religion is profoundly feminine. To begin the processes of reconstruction and restoration of the sacred feminine in Cherokee scholarship, James employs Erich Neumann's model of the Archetypal Feminine complex of the psyche, through which early humanity is related to female deities, nature, and animals at a primary level of consciousness. This model, and through it, a critical examination of Cherokee myth and its interpretations, complements the service-delivery model of Eduardo Duran inasmuch as it adds to dream theory other archetypal expressions of religious experience. Furthermore, in dealing with specific positive and negative structures of thought and emotion, it offers to the therapeutic situation a way to recognize and validate negative ecstatic experience, as found in addictive behaviors such as violence and chemical abuse. Ultimately, James argues, healing and identity for metaphysically oriented peoples must be embraced at a foundational level of mind, heart, and spirit. And depth psychology, in concert with other disciplines, gives unique access into the inherited consciousness of the Cherokee.

This chapter is particularly challenging and requires review as it attempts to address why the sacred feminine seems to have been overshadowed in recent centuries by the influence of men. At a recent symposium in Cherokee on Henry Timberlake's visit in the mid-1700s, two Cherokee scholars elaborated on the *missing* record of women's involvement in Cherokee-European contact. It was concluded that with few caveats, by the 1750s Cherokee men had learned that women were not highly regarded in trade and politics because the European system and mind-set did not condone it. And even though histories such as *Cherokee Women* by Theda Perdue (1998) and *Cherokee Women in Crisis* by Carolyn Ross Johnston (2003) have provided important information regarding how women dealt with the social, political, and cultural change of assimilation, these works do not take up the challenge of tracing women throughout the mythology and beliefs of the Cherokee and their Iroquoian predecessors to note the impact of the *absence* of the sacred feminine in contemporary society. A better understanding of women's centrality to Cherokee culture just prior to and at Contact is essential. The Cherokee have been influenced by over five hundred years of patriarchy and must deal with its residual effects, including the very real and serious contemporary social issue of violence against women.

In this text, we hope to provide readers with a broad understanding of the issues regarding Native health. By providing insight into the Cherokee perspective of health, wellness, and the end of the life cycle, one can appreciate the diversity of approaches in working with one southeastern tribal culture. Protocol and language are essential to understanding the rich variety of southeastern Indian cultures. Interestingly, hundreds of health care and service providers have been working in these communities for many years without this vital knowledge. Is it any wonder that service and provider issues in many of these communities remain problematic?

As more Cherokee and other southeastern tribal youth seek and obtain professional training in various health fields, there is hope that combined with their tribal knowledge, many of these issues will be resolved. But until then, those who work with and among tribal peoples must take the necessary steps to familiarize themselves with the perspective of the people with whom they are working. We hope this volume will be one of many that will facilitate that end.

# 1
# *Tõhi:*
## The Cherokee Concept of Well-Being

*Heidi M. Altman and Thomas N. Belt*

Encounters between Euro- and Native Americans from the earliest times have prompted individuals on both sides to marvel at the difference in languages and to wonder about the differences in ideas and perspectives that must surely follow. Nowhere have these differences drawn more interest and speculation than in the complex realm of healing and medicine. Since the period of earliest contact between Cherokees and European colonists, the distinctive features of the Cherokee medical system and beliefs have been duly noted. From Adair and Timberlake to Mooney and Olbrechts to the Kilpatricks and Fogelson, interested observers have described and documented the beliefs, practices, and formulas that form the basis of Cherokee medical practice. The Cherokee medical formulas collected and examined over the years reveal substantial portions of the ideology that underpins Cherokee healing practices. The goal of this chapter is not to add another layer of understanding to Cherokee medical practice specifically, but rather to look at the linguistic evidence for an understanding of the basic state of nature and the cosmos in the Cherokee worldview. This fundamental project will cast additional light on the materials collected by others and form the foundation for a linguistically based examination of the Cherokee medical system as it is understood today.

## Background: Challenges to Studying Cherokee Medicine

Despite the number of formulas and practices collected by various scholars, it is safe to say that there is not any one collection that adequately captures the Cherokee medical system in its entirety, especially given the individualistic nature of practitioners and their specialization in different domains of healing. As Cherokee medicine is practiced today, different types of injury or illness have their own proper means of healing (as one would expect), and practitioners tend to have a focused set of healing knowledge that pertains to a few types of injury or illness (e.g., some are adept at healing wounds from metal, others from wood; some at "working on" gastrointestinal disorders, others at respiratory disorders). Rarely if ever does one individual claim knowledge of the complete system. Rather, a practitioner will refer patients to other healers if the condition at hand is not within the realm of his or her specialty.

Historic evidence exists for the specialization of Cherokee medical practitioners in some of the earliest documentation of Cherokee and colonial government relations, dating from the early 1750s. In the South Carolina Indian Books, a collection of colonial-era papers that reflect interactions between the government of South Carolina and the native peoples of the area, one of the warriors of Settico who has interaction with the governor is known simply as "The Smallpox Conjuror of Settico." This name is used in the time period immediately following the smallpox epidemic(s) of 1736–38 that decimated the Cherokee population by half, as described by Adair. Adair's *History of the American Indians* (1930) is one of the earliest documents of the lifeways of native peoples in the Southeast. Although many of the descriptions are biased by Adair's colonial perspective and religious beliefs, they do provide some basic information about the beliefs and behaviors of the peoples he encountered. He also provides accounts of various verifiable events of the time, like the smallpox epidemics that raged through the region, from firsthand experience. The Smallpox Conjuror of Settico must have developed either a method for dealing with smallpox or been thought to have done so by enough people that he gained the appellation. From the name we can assume only that he was someone who "worked on" smallpox particularly, and presumably successfully.

An interesting perspective on the specialization of Cherokee healing is presented by Mooney in an early (1890) article in which he criticizes both prevailing notions of Indian medicine at the time and Cherokee healers themselves. Mooney points out that, as opposed to popular opinion at the time, Cherokee practitioners were not familiar with all the plants in the forest and were so specialized in their knowledge that no individual had plant knowledge greater than three hundred species—in comparison to the probable two thousand species of plants that grow in the mountain region. Interestingly, the total number of plants recognized by healers as a group was about eight hundred species or nearly half the possible total. The main thrust of Mooney's argument is that individual Cherokee healers of his time were largely ignorant of the plant species in their environment, except as they pertained to particular injuries or illnesses, and that even when a healer selected a variety of plants for healing, only one in ten had actual medicinal use. By emphasizing the circumscribed nature of Cherokee medical practice, Mooney unintentionally shows the specialization of Cherokee doctors. Over time, as we know from his later publications such as the Swimmer Manuscript, Mooney's opinions on Cherokee medicine were mitigated to some extent by his observations of practitioners at work, and he developed broader perspectives on other aspects of the healing system. However, his note about individual healers' knowledge in comparison to healers as a group, and in comparison to the knowledge of Western botanists, does show the specialization of knowledge among individual practitioners.

Specialization is also noted by Fogelson (1961), who found in his fieldwork that conjuring in general was practiced by individuals with skills pertaining to different medical conditions, as well as by individuals with skills in "ballgame conjuring, love magic, divination for lost objects," and other specialties. In fact, he points out that one of his contacts explained Will West Long's inability to cure illness, despite his extensive knowledge, as being related to his failure to specialize in one set of illnesses.

Further fragmenting a complete picture of the Cherokee medical system, individual practices are closely protected by healers and rightly valued as irreplaceable. In the past Cherokee medicine people wrote out their formulas in the Cherokee syllabary in notebooks to aid their memory in the practice of healing. The formula book of any one healer often contained his or her complete repertoire of words and actions designed to care for his or her patients. The notebooks were kept over the span of the healer's practice and some contained dozens of formulas.

Since at least the turn of the last century the notebooks have been sought for study by scholars and often have been seen as the key to understanding Cherokee medicine. Mooney, Olbrechts, Jack and Anna Kilpatrick, and Alan Kilpatrick all have produced scholarship on the available notebooks, translating the formulas and documenting the belief system. Paradoxically, however, this type of scholarship—especially the translation of Cherokee medicinal formulas into English—is thought to rob them of their power, while at the same time the Cherokee language used in many of the formulas is largely archaic, metaphorical, euphemistic, at times purposely obscure, and otherwise difficult to translate, even for native speakers (and of the list above, only the elder Kilpatricks were Cherokee speakers). In the Cherokee view, despite—or perhaps because of its very nature—the use of the language of the formulas itself enacts healing power because that language is viewed a sacred gift from the Creator. This sacred view of the language is evident in the proper Cherokee names for formulas. There are three basic names for this kind of medicine: first is *nvwoti kane:sdi* ("spoken medicine"), which indicates that simply speaking certain of the formulas is in itself a spiritual act; mere use of language accomplishes the intended practice. The second word, *nvwotiya* ("complete" or "full medicine"), refers to the words and acts. The third word, *didon(a)ti* ("the act of forcing something flexible down to the ground" [plural instances]), refers metaphorically to the power of certain medical formulas to knock a person down, or to kill him. The last type indicates the power of particular types of Cherokee medicine and the reason that translating or diverging from the proper use of the language for healing is considered an act of profanity that can render the formulas themselves ineffective. For example, the formulas and prescriptions published by Mooney and Olbrechts (1932) and by Alan Kilpatrick (1997) are considered useless by the majority of Cherokee traditionalists now that they have been translated and made widely available.

Aside from the language of the formula books, the use and handling of the books by non-trained practitioners is controversial in Cherokee communities. The means by which these books have come to be in the possession of someone other than the person who wrote the formulas in his or her own hand is always questioned, as is the intent of the person who currently possesses them. The healers themselves, who originally wrote the notebooks, may have taught, bought, sold, or traded individual formulas with other healers, but only those who were trained in the special language of and acts specified in the formulas could make use of them. Once the original practitioner is not in possession of the notebook—unless he or she has passed the notebook on to someone with special training—the notebook becomes at once useless and possibly dangerous if used by someone with improper intent. Given the possibility to effect action through words, and the possibility of "knocking a person down," it seems wise to treat these materials with all conceivable respect.

With the concerns attendant to examining the few healers' notebooks that still exist and the fewer that are available for study, we decided to approach our examination of Cherokee medicine from a different perspective. Indeed, rather than looking at illness and healing as entities separate from the rest of social life, we are interested in a holistic understanding of the neutral state of being from which illness is a departure. By clarifying the normal state of being we present a narrative context in which already recorded notions of healing and wellness can be understood. In addition, historical documents that describe reactions to and treatment practices for various epidemics can be reevaluated to gain a more complete understanding of the perspectives of Cherokee people experiencing epidemic illness. To that end we discuss here two Cherokee concepts central to the normal state of being. The first is the concept of *tōhi:*, the proper or normal state of the world, and the second is the concept of *oshi* or *osi,* the normal or neutral state of the individual.

## Methods

This research is based on verbal interviews with individuals, dictionary searches, and the analysis and correlation of information derived from both. As a native speaker of Cherokee and a university language teacher, Thomas Belt has a particular interest in and ability for analyzing Cherokee language at fundamental levels, and therefore his participation in this work was essential. As we began discussing the issue of healing and medicine we focused on the two concepts (*tōhi:* and *osi*) because they occur both in common greetings and as morphemes that indicate a state of being. Using the Cherokee Online Dictionary database (a resource developed as a collaborative project initiated by Martha J. Macri at the University of California–Davis and continued by Heidi Altman through Georgia Southern University), we were able to search information digitally scanned from various published Cherokee dictionaries and compare over five thousand lexical items from various sources and dialects. We searched for instances of these two morphemes to understand all of the ways they could be used to indicate something about the state of being in Cherokee. Additional speakers were consulted about the appropriateness of the lexical items that we compiled.

## *Tōhi:* and *Osi*

The principles established through the analysis of these two morphemes and all of the contexts in which they occur allow us to construct a model for understanding the basic workings of the world in the Cherokee view. In this section we show the ways in which *tōhi:* and *osi* can be used to indicate a proper state of being, and in the next we describe how illness is a deviation from that state.

To begin this discussion we must look at how humans are positioned in the Cherokee universe. In the Cherokee cosmology humans are considered to be anomalous, stuck in the midst of supernatural plants, animals, and other beings; guests in a complex spirit world. The spirit animals and plants have a history of their own before humans are introduced and the role of humans in the universe is that of odd pieces that must fit themselves into an already functioning whole. Cherokee oral tradition (and Cherokee mythology as published in Mooney [1900] 1992) includes a variety of stories about spirit animals and their relationship to humans, but the one that best reflects the position of humans in relation to the spirit animals is the one Mooney calls "The Origin of Disease and Medicine." In this story, humans begin to overpopulate and crowd the animals, and then slaughter them for food and step on the smaller creatures. In revenge the animals create a host of illnesses to thin the number of humans. Meanwhile, the plants, which coexist well with humans, create a remedy for every affliction the animals create.

In order to manage and maintain their position in this system, which is also populated by other spirit beings that hold unpredictable attitudes toward them, humans must observe a system of natural laws instilled through oral tradition, balance themselves among their antagonists and protagonists, and preserve a neutral position. Under this code of behavior free will is essential; the individual must choose between right and wrong action; however, there are consequences for each. Right action means that the flow of the universe will continue in the proper way; consequences for wrong action can occur in the distant future, which makes them difficult to attribute to the source wrong action, but they always occur. Tom Belt remembers as a young person seeing his father and other older men examining the newspapers and ascribing current events to the outcomes of past wrongs. The idea of consequences for past wrongs developing into contemporary problems is one of the foundation principles of Cherokee medicine. Although this concept is sometimes portrayed as superstition or magical thinking about sorcery in Mooney and Olbrechts (1932), it reflects a deeply held belief in right and wrong and a philosophical orientation toward the consequences for each—a sort of morally grounded, metaphysical, indigenous chaos theory. Metaphorically, wrong action can be seen as causing a ripple in a pond that ultimately affects everything in the pond—sometimes causing illness for individuals, sometimes causing destruction for all.

The normal state of the Cherokee universe is described as being *tōhi:*—smoothly flowing, evenly and moderately paced, fluid, and peaceful. This is thought of as the way in which grass grows and clouds move on a spring day, and the way in which things are done when they are done properly. According to Thomas Belt, *tōhi:* means "not tense, not rushed, not agitated,

Table 1.1 Occupations or Activities Inflected with *Tōhi:*

| Cherokee | Gloss |
| --- | --- |
| di ga hni do hi (or) go we li | mailman |
| a ya to hi hi | deacon; one that allots or disseminates; he is the apportioner, distributor |
| a da ti hni do hi | escort; one that leads; he will lead you around |
| di da ti hni do hi | captain, coach, steward (implies plural objects) |
| di gv no sv hi do hi | janitor |
| di ka no wa di do hi | angel |
| ga na ka ti a sde lv hi do hi | nurse |
| ga nv ta ni do hi | salesman |
| a da hwa tv hi do hi | visitor |
| a da nv te li do hi | manager |

your body's not working hard, and everything's flowing smoothly. There is no speed to it. Speed in the Cherokee world or doing things quickly means that there is a purpose or immediacy. There's no rush [implied by *tōhi:*]. . . . There is fluidity, an even steady fluidity in life, health and movement." To deviate from *tōhi:* means to hurry, to stop regularly occurring action, to take action that causes the fluidity to disperse, or to encounter obstacles. As an ideal state of being *tōhi:* can be difficult to maintain, and there are a variety of ways for this fluidity to be disrupted, including illness, aggravation, and simply being out of sorts or *nohsana.*

Morphologically *tōhi:* can be a suffix, a stem, or a free morpheme. As a suffix, *tōhi:* can be an inflectional morpheme affixed to verbs to indicate an agent who ensures that the action referred to is done right, properly or consistently. Table 1.1 illustrates several of the terms for entities (usually people) who do various tasks and to which −*tōhi:* (or -*dōhi*) is added as a suffix.

As a stem *tōhi:* can be derived (e.g., *utōhi* [a noun]) to indicate "someone who is particularly adept" at an activity. *Tōhi:* can also be the basis for the adjective *utōhi yu* (also pronounced *udōhiyu* or *dōhiyu*), which indicates that something is certain or true. The most commonly known noun of which *tōhi:* is a part is *nvkwh tōhi: yadv,* which is glossed variously as peace, health, well-being, and harmony. All of these glosses describe the underlying aspects of the condition of the universe, which in the morphological analysis of the phrase becomes clearer.

*nvkwh* (gloss unclear, but probably "now" phonologically transformed from
  *nogwu*)
*tōhi:* (fluid, flowing, easy, peaceful)
*ya* (epenthetic y + "a" present tense)
*dv* (focus marker)


Taken together these morphemes indicate that "at this present moment
things are fluid, peaceful and easy" with the implied understanding that this
is easily changeable. The changeable nature of the state of *tōhi:* is reflected
in its common use in the greeting "Tōhi-tsu," which literally means "Are
things fluid, peaceful, and easy?" This phrase is most often glossed in English textbooks, dictionaries, and conversation as "How are you?" In reality,
however, upon examination it becomes clear that there is some degree of in-
terference from English in the translation and interpretation of this phrase.
In a community where many speakers are often second-language learners,
"Tōhi gwa tsu?" is frequently assigned the same sense as the English phrase
even though there is no reference to person in the Cherokee. First-language
Cherokee speakers recognize that this phrase has additional levels of meaning and use its variants to indicate slightly different questions and in reply
provide different responses. It is possible to answer the question properly
with a variety of answers (discussed below) that reflect its deeper meaning.
However, most people answer simply "Tōhi gwu" and mean "Just fine."

In the North Carolina Cherokee communities today it is estimated that
there are fewer than 500 speakers in a resident population of nearly 8,000.
The total enrolled population of over 13,000 includes members who live
away from the communities and are less likely to be fluent speakers. "Tōhi-
tsu?" and "Osi gwa tsu?" are used regularly when speakers come into contact with each other, either at public gatherings or in private. As a form
of greeting, these are second only to "Osiyo" (or *shiyo;* "hello"), which is
said by nearly everyone upon meeting. The persistence of the *tōhi:-* and
*osi-*based greetings among fluent speakers reflects the continuation of an
ancient worldview and perspective on the Cherokee state of being. Fluent speakers, a group which not surprisingly overlaps to a large extent with
those who rely on and practice traditional medicine, consider their health
and well-being with a Cherokee-language-based perspective. The use of
these greetings among second-language learners is, in many ways, a simple
substitution for English-language-based Western concepts of greeting. The
simple substitution of words and concepts from one language for those of
another is an artifact of the language revitalization/language learning pro-

cess. To a large extent the documentation of the Cherokee language has been relatively superficial, a condition reflected by the nature of most Cherokee dictionaries. No documentary source includes in-depth semantic analysis of the concepts expressed through complex Cherokee verbs; most are simply glossaries or word lists, with the one exception being Feeling and Pulte's dictionary (1975). Even in that source, however, the format is a reflection of the time in which it was produced and the enormity of the undertaking to document even the most practical aspects of Cherokee grammar. Current projects under way by the authors of this chapter include work on a hermeneutically based dictionary that seeks to provide a rich analysis of verbs in addition to the practical pedagogical information useful to language learners.

Just as *tōhi:* refers to the state of being of the world, Cherokee speakers also use the word *osi* to refer to the proper or neutral state of the individual. In the traditional Cherokee view, the individual should be poised on a single point of balance, centered, upright, and facing forward. The dichotomy of good/bad is not actually part of the concept, but rather a central point of being is preferred. As with *tōhi:, osi* is used in the greeting "Osi gwa tsu?" And just as with *tōhi:, osi* is frequently assigned a simplified English translation. *Osi* is translated in various dictionaries as "fine" or "just fine," again reflecting the limiting effect of translation on complex concepts. The greeting is usually understood in common use as "Are you good?" while the question is more properly glossed "Are things still neutral/normal," indicating that the natural or appropriate state of being is neither good nor bad but somewhere in the middle. As with *tōhi:,* however, fluent speakers recognize that "Osi gwv tsu" as a greeting indicates an inquiry as to one's state of being. In addition, *osi* is the root for the word *osiyo,* which is commonly translated as "hello," and the root for *osda* or "good." More properly translated, *osiyo* would mean something closer to "all is normal presently" and *osda,* "normal + right now."

Using the dictionary database prompted us to take a fascinating etymological side trip that illuminated additional definitions for *osi* in the widely used dictionary prepared by Feeling and Pulte (1975). Feeling glosses *osi* as "stove." In addition, an electronic dictionary file attributed to Robert Ward glosses *osi adasdadi'i* as "stove." In discussing the translations of these words, Thomas Belt remembered that both were expressions that older people in Oklahoma had used for stove. As we talked about this over several months, Belt remembered hearing people use the word *osi* to refer to something else as well. The original *osi* structures, as Tom recalls hearing his father and another elder discuss, were individual isolation huts built of wattle and daub near the home, with a permanent fire burning inside. The *osi* was designed to provide an individual with a place to isolate him- or herself for a variety of reasons. Belt says that *osi* were for women or men in need of a period of solitude for doctoring, childbirth in the winter months, or self-isolation when an individual felt out of sorts (*nohsana*). An individual could spend time getting back to a neutral state of being by sleeping overnight in the *osi*. The *osi* was a North Carolina Cherokee structure, different in form and purpose from the sweat lodges of the Plains. In fact, while there are street names that indicate the existence of Indian hot houses or *osi* on the Qualla Boundary, at least at some time in the past, Tom says that his father and the other man who discussed the existence and purpose of *osi* did not build one in Oklahoma because they thought it would be inappropriate to do so, given their limited knowledge and experience with the structures. So, while the *osi* appears to have been an indigenous Cherokee, or at least southeastern, structure, after the disruption of the Removal it was lost to those in Oklahoma and has apparently fallen out of use in North Carolina as well.

In looking for additional sources that discussed the *osi* we also consulted Mooney and Olbrechts. Looking for the word *osi* we located it in the various chapters on women's illnesses, childbirth, and menstruation. In this context Olbrechts mentions the *osi* (1932, 123), which he asserts are menstrual lodges where women might also go for the process of childbirth and for a period of isolation after childbirth. By the time of Olbrechts's visit, however, childbirth was primarily accomplished in the house, and the *osi* had fallen from use. It seems likely that Olbrechts interpreted the *osi* of the past as menstrual lodges because he asked healers specifically about menstrual lodges and they were presented in that context. However, it is surprising that Olbrechts made no apparent connection between the *osi* (he represents it "ɔsi") and an extensive description Mooney made of what he represented as "âsi." Drawing from Mooney's field notes gathered in the 1880s, Olbrechts explains the process of undergoing a sweat bath in what Mooney called an "âsi" or hothouse. According to Olbrechts, Mooney's notes say that the "âsi" was

> a small, low hut, intended for sleeping purposes, in which a fire was always kept burning. It has but one small door, which was closed during the operation, in order to confine the steam. The patient divested himself of all clothing, and entered the "âsi," when the doctor poured the liquid over the heated stones already placed inside, then retired

and closed the door, leaving the patient to remain inside until in a profuse perspiration from the steam which filled the hothouse. The door was then opened and the man came out, naked as he was, and plunged into the neighboring stream.... The sweat bath is still in use among them, but as the "âsi" is no longer built, the patient is steamed in his own house, and afterwards plunges into the nearest stream, or is placed in the open doorway and drenched with cold water over his naked body. (61)

Despite the fact that Olbrechts did not draw a correlation between "ɔsi" and "âsi," phonetically the representations are close enough to have conceivably been the same word heard by different transcriptionists forty or more years apart. Taken together, the *osi* or healing structure Thomas Belt remembers hearing described by elders in Oklahoma, the "ɔsi" described as a menstrual lodge by Olbrechts, and the "âsi" described as an individual hothouse or sweat bath by Mooney confirm that there was, in fact, an indigenous Cherokee structure dedicated to healing that featured an always burning fire inside.

Today, the word *osi* is an apparent semantic extension used first to refer to outdoor kitchens, then to outdoor ovens that resembled the *osi* structures, then to indoor stoves or ranges. The relationship between *osi* as a neutral state of being and *osi* as a place to go to regain a neutral state of being requires some interpretation, but given the relatedness of the concepts it is not hard to imagine that in order to regain a sense of *osi,* one should spend some time in an *osi.*

## Deviation from *Tōhi:* or *Osi:* States of Imbalance or Illness

In examining the occurrence of illness in the Cherokee view, it is necessary first to understand that within the category of illness or imbalance an individual can have experiences related to his or her own actions, or those related to the actions of someone else, either of which can disrupt their own ongoing fluidity or push them out of their proper state of neutrality. Although an individual can become ill either through his or her own actions or through the actions of another, in either case the natural human condition is disrupted, sometimes resulting in overt, observable physical symptoms, and sometimes in what we might call emotional or affective symptoms. In either case the person afflicted with the anomalous condition is seen as being beset by agents who have different methods and purposes for making the individual sick. Healers collect information about the patient in general to determine the nature of the illness and sometimes, more important, the nature of its cause.

In its general sense, a disease of the body is referred to as *ahyugi* ("an angry or resentful entity that comes to visit"). When one is referring to a person who has a chronic illness or an illness that stays, the term for illness is *uwehi* ("illness that lives in the body"). In the first instance the characteristic of resentment or anger as a component of illness metaphorically reflects the story of the origin of disease and medicine as outlined above. In this context disease is sent as an expression of the anger or resentment of the spirit animals to knock humans down. In a more immediate sense, however, this is an indication of the nature of consequences for wrong acts. When one deviates from appropriate behavior, the consequence can be *ahyugi*, metaphysically speaking, the resentful act of a living cosmos, or it can be something sent to the afflicted person by another who bears resentment or anger. In any case, intention on the part of the afflicted person and the illness is crucial to understanding a proper course of treatment.

When referring to a person afflicted with a specific chronic illness, the word *uwehi* indicates that illness is an entity that has taken up residence inside the patient, again reflecting the agency of the illness, although not necessarily with the same metaphorical antecedents or intention as *ahyugi*. A person may have any of a number of different *uwehi*, including, for example, cancer *adahyesgi* ("the thing that eats a flexible object [the inanimate object classification for humans]") or tuberculosis *usihwasgv uwehi* ("coughing sickness"). More acute illnesses like the common cold are thought of as *uniyihv* ("something that grabs someone"). A sick person is referred to as *utlvga* (OK) or *utsvga* (NC). A list of words related to illness or deviation from the states of *tōhi:* or *osi* is presented in table 1.2.

In addition to diseases of the body with overt observable symptoms, individuals may experience the feeling that they are *nohsana*. This emotional or perceived state can be the result of wrong past action, or it can be an understanding that some other consequence is about to come to bear. When one feels a premonition of bad things to come, one says "Agwohiyu nohsana yigesesdi," or "I think that it will not turn out well in the future." This can be an answer in reply to "Tōhi gwv tsu," or it can be something said in general. In addition, a person can feel that another person is taking spiritual action against him or her, in which case one could answer the question "Tōhi gwv tsu" by saying "kilogohusdi nagwvneha" ("someone is making my state of being a certain way"). This is a euphemism for conjuring that reflects the notion of having one's normal state of being manipulated and al-

Table 1.2 Words Related to Illness and Deviation from the State of *Tōhi:* or *Osi*

| Cherokee | English gloss |
|---|---|
| ahyugi; or vyugi | disease; an entity that comes to visit (mentioned in Mooney and Olbrechts 1932) |
| uwehi | disease that lives in the body (literally "third person + lives + inside") |
| uniyi | he/she/it grabbed him/her/it (refers to certain types of acute illnesses) |
| duniyitani | he/she grabbed more than one with both hands (refers to certain types of acute illnesses) |
| nohsana | headed in a bad way, not appropriate, not right, out of sorts |
| agwohiyu nohsana yigesesdi | I think that it will not turn out well in the future. |
| agwadan(a)hta | my feeling(s) at present; also my thought(s) |
| ulihelisdi | ecstatic |
| unegihlita | repulsive; nasty; disgusting |
| gola ehi | pneumonia ("it lives in winter") |
| utlvga (OK) | he/she/it is sick |
| utsvga (NC) | he/she/it is sick |
| adawehi | supernatural entity or a human possessed of supernatural skill or ability |
| didon(a)ti | the act of forcefully putting a flexible object on the ground (plural instances); metaphorically refers to killing humans; the general term for formulas that accomplish this |
| adonisgi | the person who performs didon(a)ti |
| adlvstoti | to make ill |

tered by another person. This phrase would only be used among friends in a very general way to indicate this concern. If it were determined that this was in fact happening, other actions and words would be used to discuss and counter the activity. It is not permissible to translate or represent those words and actions here. If it were known, however, that a person had been made sick by conjuring or victimized by conjuring, he or she could be referred to as *atsinanesvele'i*, which has the sense of something being made impure, polluted, or contaminated. Only through ceremonial cleansing is there the possibility for healing.

## Conclusion

Although this is a brief overview of a topic that could properly fill a volume or more, we have shown that there are two related concepts that form the foundation of the Cherokee worldview. Taken together, these concepts— *tōhi:* and *osi*—indicate that there is a normal state of being for the Cherokee world and for the Cherokee individual. The Cherokee world should be fluid, peaceful, and easy like water flowing—a central feature of Cherokee country and a central component to Cherokee healing and spiritual ceremony. The proper state of the Cherokee individual is centered, balanced, and neutral—a rock with the stream of life flowing around it. When an individual does something to deviate from the state of *tōhi:* or becomes decentered, illness or other consequences can beset them. Whether the flow has been disrupted or the individual has become unbalanced, conditions are ripe for damage to self or community, and only by engaging in healing that restores the world and the individual to the appropriate state can things be made right again.

# 2
# The Unintended Consequences of Prehistoric Skeletal Studies to Modern Cherokee Communities

*Michelle D. Hamilton and Russell G. Townsend*

While anthropologists have long conducted research among the Cherokee people, many are unaware of the potential side effects to Cherokees resulting from osteological studies. Employing an emic perspective, we offer insight into the challenges posed to modern Cherokees as a result of anthropological skeletal analyses, and detail the detrimental effects to health as a result of such studies.

## Anthropology in Cherokee Country

Anthropological studies focusing on topics such as mortuary patterning, craniometric analysis, and paleopathology are not new practices in Cherokee country, having their origins in the late nineteenth century when early researchers such as Cyrus Thomas and Samuel Morton initiated scientific surveys of the mound-building peoples of the American Southeast.

Initially, Cherokee town sites did not receive the same level of scientific scrutiny as lowland mound sites because of the size, scope, and relative ease of access in the Southeast, compared to the difficulty of working in the mountainous southern Appalachian highlands.

Many Cherokee town sites occupy the same locations as Mississippian mound sites, having been built on top of them. While the majority of past archaeological research has focused on the Mississippian period, there has recently been a consistent and growing trend of interest in archaeology that relates purely to the protohistoric and historic Cherokee.

In fact, some of the largest archaeological projects in the American Southeast have focused on Cherokee town sites and their likely precursors. The Tellico Project is one such example, with excavations conducted at no fewer than ten Cherokee towns along the Little Tennessee River. While much of the research emphasis focused on developing an understanding of the late Mississippian Dallas phase people—the population that is potentially the modern Cherokee antecedent—additional effort was also directed at clarifying the historic Cherokee occupations of these sites (Chapman 1985; Polhemus 1987; Schroedl 1986).

Additional archaeological work has been done on the Mississippian and historic towns along the Hiwassee River and its drainages, including several town sites known to be occupied by the Overhill Cherokee, such as Hiwassee Old Town and Hiwassee Island. Lewis and Kneberg first undertook this work during the Works Progress Administration projects of the 1930s. Subsequent work in this vicinity has focused on trying to understand the relationship of the Mouse Creek phase to the nearly contemporary Lamar and Dallas phases, as well as the relationships of these three late Mississippian phases to the Overhill Cherokee occupation of this region (Sullivan 1987).

On the eastern side of the mountains research has been more sporadic, owing to the more mountainous terrain of the area. Excavations of a limited nature have occurred in the Tuckasiegee, Valley, Oconaluftee, Little Tennessee, and Hiwassee River valleys. Several ambitious archaeological projects have occurred in this region, including the well-known excavations at Garden Creek and the Peachtree site (Sullivan and Prezzano 2001). Again, work in the region has focused on Mississippian mound centers with research into their Cherokee occupations coming as almost a second thought.

All of these excavations contained an element of mortuary studies and skeletal biological studies, and thousands of graves were excavated at these sites. In the Tellico Project, at the town of Toqua alone more than four hundred burials were excavated. Thousands of these skeletons recovered during the Tellico Project still remain shelved in university museum storage, having received only cursory examination. Only about one hundred skeletons from the thousands recovered were identified as Cherokee, and they were reburied in 1986 at the Sequoyah Birthplace Museum in Vonore, Tennessee.

Bioarchaeologists have shown that analyzing the human skeleton is the most useful method for understanding the biological status of early human populations. Studies of mortality and morbidity in American Indian skeletal remains are an integral facet of bioarchaeological studies. People are known by the traces they leave in their passing: cultural artifacts, habitation sites, art works, and the most tangible evidence of all for their existence—their bones. The skeleton gives direct testimony of sickness, disease, nutrition, and pathologies, and allows anthropologists to reconstruct past biological histories in ways and details that other avenues of anthropological inquiry simply cannot. The insight gained from bioarchaeological examination of the skeleton allows the charting of a people's successful or failed adaptation to their environment. Today, however, as the result of modern cultural resource legislation, anthropologists who study the skeletal remains of American Indians now realize they are facing a new era in which repatriation laws, such as the Native American Graves Protection and Repatriation Act (NAGPRA) are changing the practice of American anthropology.

With the passage of repatriation legislation, anthropologists have attempted to demonstrate the value of bioarchaeological studies to living people. While the value for scientific knowledge is clear, assertions that research in areas such as cranial measurements, porotic hyperostosis, stature, caries frequencies, prehistoric life expectancies, and counts of supernumerary foramina directly benefit the health of modern Indian people are not supported.

In an effort to show the value of bioarchaeological research—and hence, the necessity of disturbing American Indian dead—some anthropologists assert that the study of prehistoric American Indian bones contributes to the health of current American Indians and that information gleaned from bioarchaeological research may some day benefit the health and welfare of all living American Indians. However, it is difficult (if not impossible) to prove this in any single case or instance, despite efforts to the contrary (i.e., Landau and Steele 1996; Ubelaker and Grant 1989; Willey 1981). Anthropologists have thus far been unable to dispute the observation offered by Dr. Emery A. Johnson, former U.S. assistant surgeon general, who worked as the director of Indian Health Service for three decades: "I am not aware of any current medical diagnostic treatment or procedure that has been derived from research on . . . [American Indian] skeletal remains. Nor am I aware of any during the 34 years that I have been involved in American Indian . . . health care" (quoted in Harjo 1989).

Certainly Cherokee people have a great interest in understanding their past, yet many Cherokees remain unconvinced that archaeology is the best or even a good method for gaining that understanding. However, the past fifteen years have seen the Cherokee people warming slightly toward the science of archaeology. We do not believe this is a reflection of changing cultural norms within the Cherokee populace but rather of the patient work of a small number of archaeologists who have taken the time to ask the Cherokee people what they want to know about their past. Archaeologist Brett

Riggs, who worked with and for the Cherokee for a number of years, has produced a fine example using Cherokee interest in ceramic manufacture to connect modern Cherokee potters with their counterparts of the past. Riggs has been able to answer the questions of interested Cherokees about the development of Qualla pottery and in doing so has fired the imagination of a new generation of Cherokee potters who once again continue the development of the Qualla tradition.

On the other hand, mortuary archaeology and studies in bioarchaeology have thus far yielded little of interest for Cherokee people. For a time mortuary patterning appeared as though it might help delineate the spatial and temporal boundaries of the Cherokee world. However, it appears that resistance to cultural resource laws like NAGPRA may have developed within the anthropological community, and archaeologists have grown reticent to use this data for affiliation purposes. With regard to skeletal biology we have yet to speak to anyone in any Cherokee community who feels these studies have contributed to their understanding of their ancestors' past. Cherokees express an understanding with regard to the lives of their ancestors and do not feel that research into diseases that troubled them or knowing average life expectancy helps them understand the past in any greater detail.

## Consequences to Health in the Living Cherokee Community

Not only has research into Cherokee skeletal biology failed to improve the health of Cherokee communities, it is believed to have done just the opposite. Traditional Cherokee beliefs hold that there are dire consequences to coming into contact with the dead without undergoing the appropriate cleansing rituals. These consequences include sickness and disease that are seen to originate from the pollution and corruption of the dead (Witthoft 1983). Great care is exercised in traditional Cherokee funerary practices, in part to avoid or cleanse participants of pollution associated with death. In addition, Fogelson indicates that besides diseases being caused by vengeful animals, sickness can also be caused by ghosts and other supernatural beings associated with death (Fogelson 1980b).

While this is not the venue to revisit discussions of these supernatural beings and it would be culturally inappropriate to do so at length, it is nevertheless important to firmly understand that Cherokees believe these supernatural creatures who spread illness and conflict are drawn to death, and this is why disease and discord are associated with proximity to the bones of the dead.

It is held by traditional Cherokees that research by anthropologists on the bones of the dead is a dire danger to the living community of modern Cherokees. These beliefs have been likened to the opinion many Americans hold toward government research into biological warfare: overarching uneasiness with regard to the government's ability to contain these experiments without causing global catastrophe. The traditional Cherokee view is nearly identical to the understanding that anyone conducting anthropological research on human remains without undergoing adequate cleansing is a carrier of disease, misfortune, and death. It is important to note that vigorously washing one's hands with hot soapy water will not do the job. Any scientist coming into Cherokee country with the intention of conducting research involving the dead is viewed as someone who will either purposefully or accidentally spread malignancy into the community. Cherokees believe that besides the introduction of malignancy, sickness, impropriety, and other malevolence, research into human remains results in additional deterioration to the health of Cherokee communities.

Numerous studies have proven the link between stress, self-esteem, and other social factors and the health status of Native Americans. These studies show that disease, infant mortality, and other factors associated with untimely death are significantly higher in communities of subjugated people (see Duran et al. 1998; Hjemdahl 2002; Joe and Young 1994; Lefler, this volume; Manson et al. 1998). Native American communities are viewed this way both within and without. Their recent history is one in which they have been decimated by war and disease, they have been forced off their land and placed in locations undesirable to Euro-American society, they are among the most poverty-stricken, they did not share the same constitutional rights as their Euro-American neighbors until eighty years ago, and the remains of their ancestors are removed from their burial grounds for the purposes of academic study. It should not be surprising that the prevalence of disease, alcoholism, and infant mortality would be higher in communities undergoing these types of chronic and acute stressors.

## Improving Relationships

Many anthropologists view themselves as interpreters of panhuman histories, including those that are not their own. This viewpoint that the ancient dead can serve to tell us about the past is undoubtedly one held by many. A conflict arises, however, when basic moral and ethical tenets of respect are violated: respect for the wishes of the dead and respect for the wishes of their descendants. Anthropologists argue that the bulk of information available on American Indian history is known by virtue of anthropological analysis, but American Indians argue that this point is arrogant and dismissive of Native American oral and cultural histories.

The continued scientific analysis of American Indian dead without express permission from their descendants is indefensible in the Cherokee worldview. Cherokees believe that disturbing the graves of a people who wanted to be placed in the ground is wrong, regardless of their lineage. The continued investigation of human remains and graves within Cherokee country is seen as yet another social injustice and, combined with other social factors, is felt to contribute to a lower health standard that affects the emotional, physical, and mental well-being of all Cherokees. Anthropologists have an obligation to the physical and spiritual well-being of a people if their research is viewed as causing grief and harm, and we advocate that anthropologists may improve their standing in Cherokee country if they consider that the future of American bioarchaeology is no longer exclusive of contemporary American Indian involvement (see Hamilton, this volume). In the case of the Cherokee people, anthropologists must consider new avenues of inquiry formed via collaborative investigations, enhancing the scientific foundations of research by also drawing on traditional Cherokee knowledge, guidance, and insight.

# 3
# Adverse Reactions
## Practicing Bioarchaeology among the Cherokee

*Michelle D. Hamilton*

> It seems from your list that you have no skull of the Cherokees. I am go-
> ing to pay them a visit about the 1st of next month and I will try to get
> you one or more if I can, but those fellows do not like that anybody dis-
> turb the bones of their dead.
> —Gerald Troost, in a letter to anthropologist Samuel Morton,
>     responding to his request for Cherokee skulls for craniometric
>     study during the 1800s (Bieder 1990, 8)

## Introduction

New and amended cultural resource legislation is changing the academic and
scientific landscape of American bioarchaeology. The ratification of the Native American Graves Protection and Repatriation Act in 1990 (NAGPRA)
was a defining event in the history of the discipline of biological anthropology, and the increasingly successful utilization of Section 106 of the National Historic Preservation Act by federally recognized sovereign tribes is
resulting in unanticipated restrictions on the collection of data from both
American Indian skeletal remains and mortuary site settings. The evolving phase in the relationship between bioarchaeologists and American Indians is examined in this context via insights provided by the Eastern Band
of Cherokee Indians.

Analyzing human bones and teeth to measure diachronic change in prehistoric populations is the most successful means of assessing past biological
and adaptive efficiency in the absence of recorded social histories. Through
the last twenty-five years of examining prehistoric human remains, biological anthropologists ("bioarchaeologists") have assembled a unique explora-
tive and ecologically based methodology, adapting techniques from traditional health sciences such as medicine, dentistry, and pathology, while
employing approaches from ancillary academic fields such as evolutionary
biology, ecology, geology, and archaeological sciences (see Armelagos, Carlson, and Van Gerven 1982; Katzenberg and Saunders 2000; Saunders and

Katzenberg 1992; Steckel 1993). The resulting body of bioarchaeological data has found increasing use in arenas outside anthropology, including economics, history, demography, geography, health, and nutrition (Coatsworth 1996; Rotberg and Rabb 1985; Steckel 1993; Steckel and Rose 2003).

For the most part, American bioarchaeologists trained prior to the millennium learned and refined their osteological skills using prehistoric American Indian skeletons from mortuary contexts for study, and the large volume of indigenous prehistoric American skeletons available for scientific analysis led to the generation of a sizable body of descriptive data for interpretation and hypothesis testing. This research resulted in the formation of cohesive ecological theories of early human biological adaptation among this continent's earliest inhabitants.

The excavation and recovery of these remains in situ from burials, mounds, tombs, inhumations, cremations, and other mortuary programs allowed the bioarchaeologist to interpret not only biological information, but cultural and social behaviors as well, leading to the development of new avenues of information regarding social status, political systems, interpersonal violence, community organization, and so forth (see Larsen 1982; Powell 1988; Storey 1992; Whittington 1997). The prehistoric North American biological and social landscape is arguably one of the world's best understood, owing in large part to bioarchaeological interpretations of that history.

As the result of recent political legislation, however, the discipline of American bioarchaeology now finds itself confronted by unanticipated legal restrictions on the scientific study and collection of data from American Indian skeletal remains. The passage of NAGPRA and enforcement of powerful cultural resource laws such as Section 106 of the National Historic Preservation Act have directly influenced the means by which American bioarchaeologists now conduct themselves and their research in North America.

These regulations now shape access and determine categories of information made available to anthropologists. To the bioarchaeological community, these regulations represent legally imposed limitations on sources of scientific information available about North America's prehistoric past. Conversely, to the American Indian community, these regulations represent overdue legal endorsement of the right to protect their own biological and cultural patrimony.

The currently evolving relationship between bioarchaeologists and American Indians can be examined by focusing on the effects of cultural legislation on both the discipline of anthropology and the culture of modern American Indian people (Baker et al. 2001). The unalterable outcome mandates that anthropologists who study American Indian skeletons must adapt their approach by creating new scientific paradigms, which draw on mutually collaborative efforts between scientists and tribal authorities.

In order to appreciate the division between the aims of bioarchaeologists and the viewpoints of American Indians, the perspective of the Eastern Band of Cherokee Indians will be presented. As a tribe, they have had and continue to have regular interaction with anthropologists on multiple levels, including ethnographic research, historical overviews, scientific analysis of their ancestral dead, retention of excavated human remains and cultural artifacts in institutional repositories, and investigation of archaeological sites (Bates 1982; Bigbee 1992; Bogan 1980; Chapman 1988, 1994; Duggan 1998; Finger 1984, 1991; Fogelson 1975; Green 1996; Howard 1997; Mooney [1891, 1900] 1992; Owsley and Bellande 1982; Owsley and Guevin 1982; Owsley and O'Brien 1982; Riggs 1999; Witthoft 1983; Wright 1974).

The Eastern Band of Cherokee Indians have a strong cultural ethos regarding mortuary behavior as well as traditionally defined and clearly elucidated restrictions toward the treatment of the dead. They are not representative of other tribal American Indian nations; in fact, they are not even representative of the other federally recognized Cherokee groups. They are a unique people formed through historical events and shaped by their own traditions, language, religion, worldview, and culture. In this respect, they are different from all other American Indian groups who also have their own diverse traditions. But they are also similar, with the same shared European contact experience, population decline, and historic treatment as other indigenous people in this country (Asad 1973; Crosby 1972; Dobyns 1976, 1983; King 1983; Lunenfeld 1991; Lurie 1988; Smith 1987; Taussig 1987; Thornton 1987, 1990; Woodward 1983). The great variety and expression of American Indian cultures existing and flourishing today in the new millennium is a testament to the perseverance of a people in the face of colonization and assimilation, and in this sense the perspectives of the Eastern Band serve as useful barometers to measure generalized American Indian perceptions toward anthropological research in Indian Country.

## The Eastern Band of Cherokee Indians

The Eastern Band of Cherokee Indians are one of only three federally recognized tribes of Cherokee Indians, along with the Cherokee Nation and the United Keetoowah Band of Cherokee, both based in Oklahoma. All three Cherokee groups trace their shared ancestry and homelands to the same regions of the southern Appalachian highlands, residing there until the majority of Cherokees were displaced to Indian Territory west of the Mississippi by President Andrew Jackson's Indian Removal Act of 1830, resulting in the infamous "Trail of Tears" (Foreman 1932; Perdue and Green 1995).

There was a group of Cherokee who avoided the Trail of Tears and the forced displacement, however. The remnants of the original populations who managed to evade removal through cunning, skill, diplomacy, and negotiation remained in western North Carolina and became the Eastern Band of Cherokee Indians (Finger 1984). In 1924, along with all other American Indians, they were finally granted U.S. citizenship with Congress's passage of the Indian Citizenship Act.

The Eastern Band of Cherokee Indians today have an enrolled membership of about 13,000, and the majority of the population (about 9,000) live in Cherokee, North Carolina, on the Qualla Boundary, which spans both Jackson and Swain counties and is composed of about 57,000 square miles of land and sits at the base of the Great Smoky Mountains National Park. The remainder of enrolled tribal members reside in nearby communities such as Snowbird in Graham County, or are dispersed throughout the United States. The Qualla Boundary is what remains of the former aboriginal homelands of the Cherokees, composed initially of ceded lands ranging over large portions of several southeastern states. In 1925 their landholdings were placed into federal trust, guaranteeing they would perpetually remain in Cherokee possession.

Today, the Eastern Band of Cherokee Indians are as modernized as any people in America and partake of all aspects of Western American culture. They are fully invested in their community, their faith, and their country. However, the Cherokee are not a completely assimilated people. Many still retain aspects of traditional culture and are committed to the maintenance of these values at both the personal level and through diverse institutions. There are a number of tribally funded departments on the Boundary devoted to traditional Cherokee culture, including linguistic programs, a granting foundation for research involving Cherokee interests in western North Carolina, the Cultural Resources Department, which is staffed with traditionalists and linguists, the Tribal Historic Preservation Office, which oversees archaeological undertakings within traditional Cherokee territory, multiple museums devoted to Cherokee culture, and sponsored celebrations, dances, children's activities, and other programs devoted to the continuance and promotion of core Cherokee values.

## Historic Beliefs Surrounding Death

To understand modern Cherokee perceptions of the dead and whether os-teological research is perceived as valuable, it is necessary to first examine historic accounts of death. Ethnographic research among the Cherokee has identified a traditional theoretical model of death structured around the "multiple souls" or "four souls" concept. John Witthoft, in an article titled "Cherokee Beliefs Concerning Death" (1983), relates information on the Cherokee four souls concept as told to him in the 1940s by Cherokee tradi-tionalist Will West Long (an informant who also worked with anthropolo-gists Leonard Broom, James Mooney, and Frank Gouldsmith Speck).

The first soul is described as that of memory and conscious life, and it is housed in the head, immediately under the intersection of the sagittal and coronal sutures of the skull ("front fontanelle," as explained to Witthoft). This soul flees the body immediately at the point of death and continues on with its own life, sometimes lingering as a benign, ghostly presence. The characteristic of this soul "is conscious, self-conscious, has personality, memory, continuity after death, and is unitary, not quantitative in its es-sence. It creates or secretes the watery fluids of the body: saliva, phlegm, cerebro-spinal fluid, lymph, and sexual fluids" (Witthoft 1983, 69). Long speculated that this soul eventually makes its way towards the west, the di-rection of the dead (u-sv-hi-yi, or the "Darkening Land"), or that this soul searched out entrances to the underworld by following paths of rivers and entering through spring-heads. Witthoft speculates the practice of scalping is intended to affect this soul. Once this soul leaves the body, the remaining three souls also begin to die.

The second soul is that of the physiology and is seated in the liver. This soul begins to leave the body at the point of death but departs in degrees, with the entire soul gone by the seventh day. The characteristic of this soul is "a substance, is not anthropomorphic in any [way], has no individuality, and is quantitative, there is more or less of it. It secretes yellow bile, black bile, gastric juice, etc." (Witthoft 1983, 69). The location of this soul in the liver is significant, as the liver is the organ especially subject to magical attack by witches who may turn the liver yellow (manifested as hepatitis or cirrho-sis) or black (manifested as gallbladder maladies or pancreatitis). The liver is prized by witches, who consume the organ to prolong their lives. Once the liver is "exhausted" by these maleficent forces, physiological death occurs as a result of the "absence of the soul" (Witthoft 1983, 69). Will West Long related the following explanation to Witthoft with reference to this soul and its attraction for witches.

> When the animating soul of conscious life leaves the body at the moment of death, stopping all life processes, the other souls begin to die. That of the liver is gradually diffused back into nature as a life-force and it takes a week for all of it to disappear from the body, if death has been normal. If death has not been caused by liver-soul loss, all of this soul is still present at death, and is available to the witch in the dying or the newly dead as an intact resource for extended life. With each day after death the resource is dwindling and is less tempting to the witch, so that the greatest danger is in the first night after death, less danger the first night after burial, and much less the second night after burial. Loss of the liver soul to the witches seems to do no damage to the first soul of the deceased or to the living community, so there is no practical reason why it should not be permitted. However, it is viewed as desecrative of the corpse, and also, attempts by witches give the opportunity to the conjuror to try and kill the witch, thus eliminating an enemy of the community who is dangerous in other contexts. The conjuror expects witch attacks at night just before death, during the first night after death, and soon after burial, and so keeps his lonely vigil just before death and just after death and after burial. The defenses against or obstacles to successful witch attacks are the strength or health of the victim, if alive, the strength and magical power of the fire on the household hearth, and the magical power, vigilance, and knowledge of the conjuror. Powerful witches will make their attempt to steal the liver-soul the first night after death and the first night after burial; only very feeble, incapable, and desperate witches would be tempted by the small residues left six days after death. The great crisis and the great magical conflicts would come the night after death, with the conjuror keeping his solitary vigil before the fireplace in the room with the corpse. (Witthoft 1983, 69–70)

The third soul is of the blood or circulation, and it is housed in the heart. This blood soul takes a month to leave the body from the point of death. Its characteristics are that it is "non-individual and quantitative . . . its substance gradually diffusing back into nature as a life force" (Witthoft 1983, 70). Unlike the liver, the organ of the heart or the blood soul itself "is of no use or interest to witches or conjurors after death. The living may be attacked by magic through the blood soul, in methods called 'blood sucking,' producing various anemic diseases" (Witthoft 1983, 70).

The fourth soul is that of the bones, and it takes a full year to dissipate from the moment of death. Like the blood soul, the bone soul also diffuses back to nature, where its byproducts are converted and it lends "its material to the growth of crystals in the ground, especially to the quartz crystals used in divination and conjuring" (Witthoft 1983, 70). Conjuring is the casting of malevolent actions or forces against an enemy via secret chants, formulas, and potions. Even today among many modern Cherokee, being conjured against is a real threat that can be countered through the use of protective medicines and magic.

Today, it is almost impossible to find retention or even recognition of the traditional four souls concept among the younger Cherokee generation. Even among the elderly population and among respected traditionalists and Cherokee elders, the concept may be recognized, but the stages are not credited as functional or practical explanations of the body's postmortem processes. Western Judeo-Christian biblical concepts of death, heaven, and hell have supplanted this traditional interpretation, with the Christian afterlife and its attendant single-soul concept the dominant belief among modern Eastern Band Cherokees (Hughes 1982).

In spite of this, a limited residual of the four souls tradition still appears to be in existence, especially as it concerns the vulnerability of the physiological soul to supernatural exploitation. Witches remain a dangerous facet of life in Cherokee country, and Cherokee stories still abound with cautionary tales of witches attempting to ingest the livers of the dead. The wake in Cherokee funerals lasts a full seven days (the period it traditionally takes the physiological soul to dissipate within the liver), and relatives or family friends sit with the body at night during the extended wake (Hughes 1982). The most vulnerable period for the soul of the dead person is the first night after death, when the liver is still nutritive and whole and when witches (tsi-sgi-li), also known as "night goers" (sv-no-yi ane-do-hi), "evil speakers" (u-ya igawa-sti), and powerful Raven Mockers (kalona a-ye-li-sgi) are most likely to seek out the liver for consumption in order to preternaturally prolong their lives.

Many past (and some contemporary) eyewitness accounts place witches and Raven Mockers at the scene of freshly disturbed graves. Witches and

Raven Mockers are not united in purpose, however. Instead, a natural hierarchy exists and witches are "jealous of the Raven Mockers and afraid to come into the same house with one. When at last a Raven Mocker dies, these other witches sometimes take revenge by digging up the body and abusing it" (Mooney [1891, 1900] 1992, 402). According to Cherokee scholar Alan Kilpatrick, the belief in these malevolent beings is very real, and "to the Cherokee sensibility witches (whether male or female) represent the ultimate expression of human depravity and antisocial deviance. This is their cardinal trait" (1997, 10). Fogelson also notes that many Cherokees view these creatures who feed from the dead as "undead" themselves because they offend Cherokee notions of order and lack morality (1979, 87).

The Cherokee, therefore, do not utilize the traditional belief in the four souls as a working conceptualization of osteological disintegration and the rationale for prohibition against bioarchaeological research. Instead, Cherokee opposition against the anthropological study of the remains of their dead stems from a complicated avoidance proscription based on cultural theories of pollution and corruption, as well as a deeper conviction that it is degenerate behavior to disturb the dead and runs counter to moral human behavior. These intertwined worldviews make up the Cherokee ethos regarding mortuary treatment of the dead, and influence attitudes and opinions toward bioarchaeological research.

The viewpoints in the next section were derived from conversations with Cherokee elders, traditionalists, and others who guide and oversee Cherokee policies concerning external anthropological/archaeological research utilizing Cherokee cultural resources. This information was collected during the course of the author's employment within the Tribal Historic Preservation Office (THPO) of the Eastern Band of Cherokee Indians (EBCI), where issues concerning excavation and scientific research of prehistoric remains were commonly addressed. Because of the culturally sensitive nature of this topic to tribal members, specific information regarding specialized Cherokee cultural beliefs about the dead that are not already printed, published, outlined, or understood from other arenas will not be disclosed (Fogelson 1975, 1979; Hughes 1982; Townsend and Hamilton 2004; Witthoft 1983). With this caveat in place, the following information is a representative overview of tribal opinion as it relates to general Cherokee perspectives on the sanctity of the dead, prohibitions against contact and proximity with the dead, perceptions of bioarchaeological research, and other central motifs making up the Cherokee worldview as it relates to this theme.

## Death as Contamination: Protecting the Living from the Dead

The topic of corpse pollution, disease, malignancy, and required purification ceremonies are culturally sensitive and private topics among the Cherokee. The majority of this section relies on previously published information to outline traditional prohibitions and the actions necessary to negate the dangerous effects of contact with the dead.

The fundamental precept of the Cherokee worldview is the concept of sustained order. This is accomplished, both by the individual and by the community, by adhering to two basic tenets, balance and purification, which are accomplished through "ethical action" and "mutual concern and mutual respect" for others (Kilpatrick 1997, 100). As Hughes reinforces, "The dichotomy of purity and pollution is the central theme in the Cherokee belief system. Nowhere is this more evident than in the beliefs concerning death. Contact with the dead through preparation of the dead for burial or attending a funeral can cause spiritual contamination, which is both harmful and contagious" (1982, 73).

Cherokee behave in culturally appropriate behaviors designed to avoid corruptive pollution from a variety of sources, chief among them the bodies of the dead. This is as true today as it was in 1775, when James Adair traveled through Cherokee country and witnessed that "the Cherokee observe this law of purity in so strict a manner, as not to touch the corpse of their nearest relation" (1930, 130). Kilpatrick relates that in historic times, in order to "restrict the spread of contamination," Cherokees preassigned individuals in the community to be responsible for the treatment and disposition of the dead (1997, 102), and indeed a Cherokee in his late forties confirmed that his own mother was once assigned this responsibility, noting that a woman in the community was chosen to attend to female deaths while a man was chosen to attend to male deaths. Another traditionalist related that many modern Cherokee still avoid visiting cemeteries and grave sites after family members have been interred.

Accidental exposure to the residue of the dead was also dangerous, as is related by an informant of Kilpatrick's parents, who advised, "when building a house one must be eternally vigilant about the materials used because blocks of sand and gravel may contain the disintegrated bodies of the dead. Even new lumber may be impregnated with the blood of the dead" (Kilpatrick 1997, 103). The dead are viewed as vessels of pollution by the Cherokee.

Traditional Cherokee beliefs hold that there are dire consequences to coming into contact with the dead without undergoing the appropriate cleansing rituals. These consequences include sickness and disease that are seen to originate from the pollution and corruption of the dead (Hughes 1982, Kilpatrick 1997, Witthoft 1982). Great care is exercised in traditional Cherokee funerary practices, in part to avoid or cleanse participants of pollution associated with death (Hughes 1982). In addition, Fogelson (1979) indicates that besides diseases being caused by vengeful animals, sickness can also be caused by ghosts and other supernatural beings associated with death. (Townsend and Hamilton 2004, 6)

This is at the heart of what Cherokee elders and traditionalists believe: negative forces are drawn to bones of the dead, and the living can become infected and spread the contagion to others. In order to cleanse and purify individuals who have come into contact with the dead, purification rituals must be performed. These involve water as a purifying and cleansing agent, and the ceremony of "going to water" (amo-hi at-sv-sdi, "to go to [the] water place"). Mooney relates the following historic account of the purification ritual: "The details of the ceremony are very elaborate and vary accordingly to the purpose for which it is performed. . . . The bather usually dips completely under the water four or seven times, but in some cases it is sufficient to pour water from the hand upon the head and breast" ([1891, 1900] 1992, 335).

Hughes, a Cherokee scholar and member of the Eastern Band, relates that even in modern times this ritual purification is still performed to protect the living from the effects of the dead and the associated dangers that come with exposure: "Today, after a funeral some family member makes sure that no one is affected by the deceased through the ritual of 'going to water.' This can be achieved either by going to a riverside, a small branch, or one can get water from the creek and put it into a small container. The Indian doctor will use the water and his abilities to foresee any dangers that lie ahead. If there is some reason to show concern the head member of the family will be told. Then a series of 'going to water' will be advised for the afflicted until the danger of being affected is cleared" (1982, 76).

Anthropologists must therefore realize the Cherokee have strongly ingrained aversions to the dead. Ultimately, bioarchaeologists who anticipate conducting research with skeletal remains in Cherokee Country must contend with is the following:

It is nevertheless important to firmly understand that Cherokees believe that supernatural creatures who spread illness and conflict are drawn to death, and this is why disease and discord are associated with proximity to the bones of the dead. It is held by traditional Cherokees that research by anthropologists on the bones of the dead is a dire danger to the living community of modern Cherokees ... anyone conducting anthropological research on human remains without undergoing cleansing is a carrier of disease, misfortune, and death. Any scientist coming into Cherokee country with the intention of conducting this research is viewed as someone coming into the community and either accidentally or purposefully spreading malignancy. (Townsend and Hamilton 2004, 6)

Cherokee outrage over the excavation and study of their ancestors' bones resonates on two levels: first, it is morally and ethically wrong to disturb the rest of the dead and is therefore unbalanced and immoral behavior; and second, the dead are extremely and potently dangerous to the living, and when anthropologists unearth and study remains they subject the Cherokee community to contamination and a host of other ill effects. Hughes sums up cultural prohibitions against contact with the dead in this way: "Among traditional Cherokees the concepts of purity and pollution regarding the dead are still prevalent. These deeply rooted ideas have survived two centuries of Christian influence. These vestiges will probably outlast all other remnants of traditional culture" (1982, 84).

## The Cherokee Doctrine of Non-Disturbance

When asked to explain what importance Cherokees place on the retention and maintenance of original burial and interment sites, a number of explanations were offered. Interestingly, all utilized themes of location, geography, and space as they related to the Cherokee cosmological model of balance. When speaking of the skeletons of their ancestors still buried, one Cherokee echoed this observation by stating, "They are still here, and if we disturb them we've upset order and balance. Once their resting place is disturbed, it's no longer sacred. Their existence   our existence—is wiped away." A Cherokee traditionalist further illustrated this tie to the sacredness and inviolability of space: "If you move Stonehenge, it becomes just another pile of big rocks. The meaning and essence is gone."

So important is the concept of non-disturbance and maintenance of balance that the official EBCI THPO *General Guidelines for the Re-Interment of*

*Native American Remains* outlines proper procedures to follow to maintain balance. The first preference of the THPO is always "preservation in place." This means avoidance of human burials through research design, creative planning, protective measures, and other methods to ensure burials are left in situ.

By an act of Tribal Council, the Eastern Band has also legislated the treatment and sanctity of buried Cherokee ancestors. Articles 1 and 2, Section 70, of the Cherokee Code (published by Order of the Tribal Council of the Eastern Band of Cherokee Indians and codified through Resolution Number 20, enacted on October 10, 2001) address "Skeletal Remains and Burial Site Preservation," and include sections of relevance to osteological research.

> *Section 70-2.* Sanctity of ancestors who are buried throughout the aboriginal Cherokee lands: The joint policy of the Tribal Council of the Cherokee Nation and the Eastern Band of Cherokee is as follows:
> (a) The graves of our ancestors are sacred and we desire that they not be disturbed.
> (b) In the event the remains of Cherokee ancestors are excavated, such remains shall be reburied together with all associated grave artifacts, as soon as shall be reasonable.
> (c) The remains of Cherokee ancestors should not be subjected to destructive skeletal analysis.
> (d) The remains of Cherokee ancestors and associated grave artifacts which have been disinterred and are now in possession of museums, universities, federal agencies or other institutions and persons, should be returned to the proper tribes for reburial.
> (e) Such remains should be buried at the original site where possible. (Resolution Number 121, 4-5-1990; Resolution Number 301, 5-29-1991).

When the Cherokee speak of "disturbing" human remains (the undeniable result of bioarchaeological excavations), Section 70 offers a legal definition for the term. It reveals a level of meaning extending into the realm of purposeful and, to the Cherokee culture, malevolent and unbalanced action: "Disturb includes defacing, mutilating, injuring, exposing, removing, destroying, desecrating, or molesting in any way."

## Cherokee Perspectives on NAGPRA and Repatriation

NAGPRA and other cultural resource laws have been employed for the benefit of tribal interests all across North America. To the Cherokee, this law is one more tool in their arsenal of heritage laws used to great effect to protect their traditions, their culture, their sovereignty, and their dead. But for the Cherokee, NAGPRA is not a perfect law, and is not without its flaws. Because the ultimate result of the concluded NAGPRA process is the return of human remains to the affiliated tribe, more often than not this means a direct transfer of human materials from the returning institution to Cherokee representatives. As has been made clear, proximity of living Cherokee to the remains of the dead is strictly avoided on the basis of cultural concerns for the health and welfare of the living, as well as the potential for them as vectors of transmission to spread contamination to the entire community. A Cherokee traditionalist explained it this way: "To give the remains back [to Cherokee people] makes us an accessory to the disturbance, to unbalance. We have to do a lot of preparation to make sure we are protected and that they [the Cherokee ancestors who are now skeletal remains] don't transfer over anything to us if we have to receive them back. That's what people didn't think about when they wrote NAGPRA."

When asked how this situation could be resolved or alleviated, he responded that because human remains are so dangerous to the Cherokee, it is better that no living Cherokee come into contact with them. The solution, in his opinion, was "for the people who had disturbed the remains already to do the right thing and rebury them—not expose us to them."

## Representations of Death in Cherokee Culture

Official written policy as outlined in the protocol document EBCI THPO "Treatment Guidelines for Human Remains and Funerary Objects (Survey, Excavation, Laboratory/Analysis, and Curation Guidelines)" includes the following statement with reference to photography of human remains: "The EBCI requests that in the event human remains, funerary objects, sacred objects, or objects of cultural patrimony are encountered, no photographs of such items be taken. Detailed drawings are permissible, however."

The Eastern Band of Cherokee Indians view photographs of the dead as actual representations of death, and photographic depictions of the dead are as hazardous to Cherokee health and well-being as exposure to actual skeletal remains. Perhaps one of the most important points for the anthropologist to realize is that Cherokee aversion to death involves clear avoidance of *all* dead, not just Cherokee dead. This extends to the dead of other American Indian groups, to African American dead, and to Euro-American dead, in short, to the dead of any member of humanity, regardless of ancestry or ethnicity.

Cherokee traditionalists and elders affirm that photographs of the dead are as potent as the actual bones of the dead, and thus are classified as objects to be avoided. The reason photographs are seen to manifest the same potentiality for disease, discord, and social unease is that digital and photographic images captured by light are perfect one-to-one depictions of death and are culturally and physically dangerous to Cherokee society in a manner that sketches, drawings, and other "imperfect" captures made by human hand and through human interpretation are not (Russell Townsend, personal communication, 2004).

## Cherokee Expectations of Anthropologists

It comes as no surprise that the overwhelming majority of archaeologists and physical anthropologists working in Indian country have been poor ambassadors for the field of anthropology. When conducting research on American Indian cultures, anthropologists enter Indian communities, examine Indian dead, research Indian history, excavate Indian sites, examine Indian documents, and interview Indian people. They collect data, transform it into a body of academic work, and often neglect to inform the American Indian community of their findings in ways accessible to the non-academic layperson. The experience of the American Indian has been that anthropologists always take but that they rarely, if ever, give back.

As a result of this apparent unwillingness or inability to disseminate the results of research gathered solely by virtue of another culture's existence, many Cherokees view anthropologists as elitists who collect information on Cherokee society and transform that knowledge into personal cachet, monetary reward, academic prestige, thesis and dissertation topics, journal and book publications, and tenure opportunities with complete disregard for the fact that Cherokees might actually wish to learn the results to potentially gain more insight as well. As Mihesuah notes, "American Indian remains, their cultural objects, in addition to their images, serve as the focal points of many anthropologists' careers. The fact that Indians exist allows these people—as well as historians—to secure jobs, tenure, promotion, merit increases, fellowships, notoriety, and scholarly identity—all without giving anything back to the Indian community" (2000, 97).

At consultation meetings between professional anthropologists and Cherokees in late 2004, the Cherokees were asked if they valued anthropological research. They responded that they would be very interested in learning the results of that research, but that it was never shared with them. This is a remarkable indictment of the unprofessional disregard anthropologists hold for native communities. The number of times anthropologists have shared their research with the Eastern Band can probably be counted on one hand, but the results have been stunning.

> Certainly Cherokee people have a great interest in understanding their past, yet many Cherokees remain unconvinced that archaeology is the best or even a good method for gaining that understanding. However, the past fifteen years have seen the Cherokee people warming slightly towards the science of archaeology. We do not believe that this is a reflection of changing cultural norms within the Cherokee populace, but rather of the patient work of a small number of archaeologists who have taken the time to ask the Cherokee people what they want to know about their past. Brett Riggs has produced a fine example using Cherokee interest in ceramic manufacture to connect modern Cherokee potters with their counterparts of the past. Dr. Riggs has been able to answer the questions of interested Cherokees about the development of Qualla pottery and in doing so has fired the imagination of a new generation of Cherokee potters who once again continue the development of the Qualla tradition. (Townsend and Hamilton 2004, 7)

However, when Cherokee elders were asked about the ultimate value of skeletal and bioarchaeological studies to the community, they were hard-pressed to find a benefit.

> Mortuary archaeology and studies in bioarchaeology have yielded little of interest for Cherokee people. For a time mortuary patterning appeared as though it might help delineate the spatial and temporal boundaries of the Cherokee world. However, as resistance to cultural resource laws like NAGPRA has developed within the anthropological community, archaeologists have grown reticent to use this data for this purpose. With regard to skeletal biology we have yet to speak to anyone in any Cherokee community who feels these studies have contributed to their understanding of their ancestors' past. (Townsend and Hamilton 2004, 7)

This stance reflects a number of missed opportunities presented to bioarchaeologists. Interaction with American Indian communities must be undertaken on an equal footing, which involves understanding the living culture even while studying its past. An awareness of the cultural sensitivities involved with types of bioarchaeological research will enhance all levels of research. Another missed opportunity is to return back to the Indian community a portion of what was taken away; the Cherokee are interested in their past and want to know the results of academic research on their people. By involving tribes in anthropological research, bioarchaeologists can change the perceptions held by many tribal groups.

Anthropological historian Bruce Trigger offers the following comment, which most members of the Eastern Band (indeed, most American Indians) would echo.

> Viewing the Indians' past as a convenient laboratory for testing general hypotheses about sociocultural development and human behavior may be simply a more intellectualized manifestation of the lack of sympathetic concern for native peoples that in the past has permitted archaeologists to disparage their cultural achievements, excavate their cemeteries, and display Indian skeletons in museums without taking thought for the feelings of living native peoples. If prehistoric archaeology is to become socially more significant, it must learn to regard the past of North America's native peoples as a subject worthy of study in its own right, rather than as a means to an end. . . . [B]y treating generalizations about human behavior as being the primary or even the only significant goal of archaeological research, archaeologists have chosen to use the data concerning the native peoples of North America for ends that have no special relevance to these people. Instead, they are employed in a clinical manner to test hypotheses that intrigue professional anthropologists and to produce knowledge that is justified as serving the broader interests of Euroamerican society. (1980, 671)

## Bioarchaeological Ethics

"Many scientific associations are beginning to reconsider ethical principles that underlie their research activities. The field of bioarchaeology is especially problematic in this respect, positioned as it is between medicine, with its ethical focus on generating scientific knowledge for use in helping individual patients, and anthropology, with its ethical principles that stem from deep belief in the power of cultural relativism to overcome ethnocentrism and encourage tolerance" (Walker 2000, 3).

Many scientific disciplines have been forced to address the ethical implications of their research, and bioarchaeology is no exception. It is uniquely situated to address the ethical and moral components of its epistemological efforts; namely, *how we come to know* must be balanced against *by what means we come to know*. This distinction is critical for a discipline that must both contend with public sentiment and depend on public funding for many of its directives and research initiatives.

What, then, is the purpose of anthropological science? Does it have responsibilities to the public good, and if so, what are they? In medical science, the Hippocratic dictum "Primum non nocere" ("First, do no harm") guides practice and research, but what moral standard guides bioarchaeologists? More than a decade after the passage of NAGPRA, the development of a "uniform set of standards for the study of human subjects, [by which] osteologists will follow the same procedures for the prehistoric dead as are now required for research on the living and the recently dead (e.g. autopsy studies)" anticipated by Rose and coworkers in their seminal paper addressing the impact of NAGPRA on osteological studies still has not come to pass (1996, 100).

The professional organization of American bioarchaeologists, the American Association of Physical Anthropologists (AAPA), includes a code of ethics for its membership, which was adopted in 2003. Nowhere in this ethics code does the AAPA specifically address issues concerning the use of American Indian skeletal remains for research, potential obligations of bioarchaeologists to descendant American Indian communities, and American Indian rights to their own biological and cultural patrimony. The section in the code that may come closest to addressing these concerns is one that discusses research on human and primate subjects.

Responsibility to people and animals with whom anthropological researchers work and whose lives and cultures they study.

1. Anthropological researchers have primary ethical obligations to the people, species, and materials they study and to the people with whom they work. These obligations can supersede the goal of seeking new knowledge, and can lead to decisions not to undertake or to discontinue a research project when the primary obligation conflicts with other responsibilities, such as those owed to sponsors or clients. These ethical obligations include:

   To respect the well-being of humans and nonhuman primates.

   To work for the long-term conservation of the archaeological, fossil, and historical records.

   To consult actively with the affected individuals or group(s), with the goal of establishing a working relationship that can be beneficial to all parties involved.

2. Anthropological researchers must do everything in their power to ensure that their research does not harm the safety, dignity, or privacy of the people with whom they work, conduct research, or perform other professional activities.

The lack of defined ethical guidelines for bioarchaeological researchers and students working with American Indian skeletal remains is disadvantageous to the discipline in a variety of academic, legal, professional, and public arenas. The AAPA includes no wording or protocols directed toward the study of American Indian dead, and it is uncertain whether specific guidelines will ever be incorporated into an ethical policy, owing to the fundamental difficulties of reconciling the goals of American bioarchaeology with the new realities of cultural resource legislation.

A number of professional anthropological (non-bioarchaeological) associations are cognizant of potential ethical dilemmas that may arise during the study of living indigenous people, their deceased ancestors, and their material culture. While most of these organizations do not outline specific guidelines for research with skeletal remains and procedures of repatriation, their statements on expected ethical behavior can be interpreted as applying to the subject in various degrees, as echoed by Garza and Powell: "Archaeologists are funded primarily from public coffers. Native Americans are a part of that public, and archaeologists must be responsive to their legitimate concerns. Many archaeologists are doing so. However, with the exception of SOPA [Society of Professional Archaeologists] and WAC [World Archaeological Congress], archaeological professional organizations do not recognize this obligation in their ethical statements" (2001, 52).

The Society for American Archaeology (SAA) is the main professional body of practicing archaeologists in the United States. Founded in 1935, the SAA has bylaws that include regulations for members on the subject of ethics as they apply to their profession, to their colleagues, and to the public. Their statement regarding the excavation and study of human remains, however, does not address the ethical implications of working with American Indian skeletal remains: "Research in archaeology, bioarchaeology, biological anthropology, and medicine depends upon respectable scholars having collections of human remains available both for replicative research and research that addresses new questions or employs new analytical techniques. . . . Whatever their ultimate disposition, all human remains should receive appropriate scientific study, and should be accessible only for legitimate scientific or educational purpose."

The Vermillion Accord on Human Remains (World Archaeological Congress 1989) outlines six tenets for working with skeletal remains of the dead.

1. Respect for the mortal remains of the dead shall be accorded to all, irrespective of origin, race, religion, nationality, custom and tradition.
2. Respect for the wishes of the dead concerning disposition shall be accorded whenever possible, reasonable and lawful, when they are known or can be reasonably inferred.
3. Respect for the wishes of the local community and of relatives or guardians of the dead shall be accorded whenever possible, reasonable and lawful.
4. Respect for the scientific research value of skeletal, mummified and other human remains (including fossil hominids) shall be accorded when such value is demonstrated to exist.
5. Agreement on the disposition of fossil, skeletal, mummified and other remains shall be reached by negotiation on the basis of mutual respect for the legitimate concerns of communities for the proper disposition of their ancestors, as well as the legitimate concerns of science and education.
6. The express recognition that the concerns of various ethnic groups, as well as those of science are legitimate and to be respected, will permit acceptable agreements to be reached and honoured.

While the Vermillion Accord does apply to the dead, its tenets have not been adopted by the AAPA. Research involving the prehistoric dead should be a subject of discussion within the bioarchaeological community and it may be useful to frame the debate by examining other scientific fields that also address ethical and moral questions concerning use of the dead for research purposes (Goldstein and Kintigh 1990; Hubert 1994; Watkins 1999).

## Invasion of the Body Snatchers

Human bodies are valuable as commercial commodities and research materials in biomedical research fields. Human tissues, including bone, are regularly subject to monetary, academic, and scientific transactions within the research community. The use of human bodies for anatomical research purposes in America has often been controversial and continues to be so today, with debate centering on lack of personal or familial consent, commercial value, and research potential.

The question of bioethics and research using bodies of the non-consenting dead (both prehistoric and modern) is a complicated issue that has received much consideration in biomedical settings. The dead body, whether fresh in a necropsy setting or hundreds of years old in an archaeological setting is classified as an "ambiguous entity"; legally recognized as having both "sacred meaning . . . [and] instrumental value as an object for scientific study, clinical teaching and commercial gain" (Nelkin and Andrews 1998, 261).

Early in the history of medicine, the dissection of the dead by anatomical researchers like Galen, Da Vinci, and Vesalius was an established practice (Sawday 1995), and by the turn of the nineteenth century, "the corpse was well-integrated in clinical thought, and the anatomical findings revealed by autopsies became the basis for both medical understanding and the development of the field of pathology" (Nelkin and Andrews 1998, 262). Despite this, the institutionalized practice of using human bodies for training, experimentation, and research had not been widely accepted by the public (Jackson 1950). Early in America's medical history, the sources from which human corpses were procured tended toward the more unsavory, including executed criminals, the homeless, and other socially marginalized members of society because in the public perception, "dissection remained a humiliation imposed on social outcasts" (Humphrey 1973, 824).

Soon, the medical demand for the dead reached proportions beyond available supply, leading to a surge of "body snatching" by medical students, who were expected to arrive at college with their own cadavers in tow, or by third-party "resurrectionists" who procured cadavers for medical colleges (Richardson 1987). Body snatching, the unearthing and theft of recently buried bodies from graveyards, became a profitable industry. Black cemeteries and potter's fields for the poor soon were looted. Demand eventually reached into cemeteries of all Euro-American social classes, fueling fears among the public that their bodies would be stolen from the grave and used for dissection and scientific research. In the 1700s, when burials at the Trinity Church in New York began to be looted by nearby Kings' College medical students, community sentiment turned to anger and fear (Heaps 1970).

By the late 1700s, Euro-American public outrage had reached a threshold. In New York a body-snatching incident in 1788 caused public mob rioting by the thousands when medical students were discovered practicing dissection on a recently dead woman known to the community. The "Doctor Riots" lasted three days, after which the students and physicians fled and sought safety in jail, where they were eventually prosecuted and fined (D. Thomas 2000). This incident resulted in the development of new laws: the Anatomy Acts of 1789 "decreed not only what bodies could be used for research but also made it legal for the courts to add dissection to the death penalty in cases of murder, arson, and burglary . . . [and] also established punishments for grave robbers" (Bieder 1990, 21). Despite these and national laws that were enacted specifically to address the shortage and regulate the use of cadavers by the medical community (allowing anatomical schools to legally utilize the bodies of the unclaimed dead for dissection), "doctors and teachers in individual states . . . still encountered difficulty in legally securing sufficient bodies, and body snatching continued in rural areas well into the 1800's" (Heaps 1970, 21).

In the modern age, of course, body snatching for medical research and clinical training is no longer practiced. The medical community gave up what was to them a lucrative method of procuring bodies for anatomical dissection—halting only when the tide of political and public opinion turned against these practices. However, this did not curtail their ability to conduct medical research. Gifts of anatomical donations by consenting individuals and state laws allowing the donation of the unclaimed dead by coroners and medical examiners ensure there are medical cadavers available for training and teaching purposes. Also exciting is the increasing use of technological methods such as three-dimensional imaging, computerized medical mannequins, and virtual simulators to hone dissection and surgical techniques previously only practiced on cadavers.

In many respects, this episode in medical history may have parallels to what is occurring today in bioarchaeology with the use of American Indian skeletal remains for research. Political and public awareness of bioarchaeologists has heightened and shifted with the enforcement of laws like NAGPRA to protect American Indian dead, and efforts to regulate anthropological research in these arenas may be a forerunner to even more pronounced social reaction and stringent legal prohibition in the future.

## Mortui Vives Docent

The use of the deceased to teach the living has an ancient and hallowed history. The corpse has served as a valuable instructor to the medical establishment, and in bioarchaeology the dead serve as guides to the past. The examination of prehistoric human skeletal remains forms the basis of all scientific research in bioarchaeology, and studying the unearthed dead to complete a picture of humanity's past "has both intrinsic and instrumental value. All humans can benefit from it, and in that sense, all humans have a stake in its acquisition" (Schrag 2002, 2).

That the ancient dead can serve to tell us about the past is not in doubt.

The conflict arises, however, when cultural norms and mores are violated during the acquisition of this knowledge, in this instance, respect for the wishes of deceased American Indians to remain buried and respect for the wishes of their descendants to ensure these remains are not disturbed and harvested for the purposes of scientific research.

Ethical conflicts for the use of American Indian skeletons by bioarchaeologists may be classified as falling under the following moral and legal rubrics, as noted by Schrag (2002):

1) lack of consent by the deceased to be used as research materials
2) custodial ownership of human remains
3) intrinsic value of bioarchaeological research
4) prejudicial treatment

These broad categories encompass many moral, legal, and scientific positions, and a brief examination will reveal that while there are no easily applied answers to clarify the debate, there are a number of considerations that must be analyzed by bioarchaeology students and researchers actively using the skeletons of non-consenting American Indians in their research.

1) *Lack of consent to be used as research materials.* What is the obligation to respect the dead if their wishes are not expressed in writing? In the case of prehistoric dead, of course, there are no written instructions; therefore, is it reasonable to assume that deliberate burial implies an express wish on the part of the individual or the group to remain undisturbed? Does the absence of written or verbal consent obviate the sanctity of the grave and indicate permission for bioarchaeologists to utilize human bodies for their own research agendas? Is bioarchaeological research automatically a matter of conscription for dead American Indians above all other ethnic groups?

When a modern individual wishes their remains to be used for medical purposes or scientific research (i.e., organ donation, medical cadavers, or anthropological studies), advance consent must first be obtained from that individual or members of the decedent's family. It would be considered morally inappropriate (and indeed illegal) to remove from hospitals, funeral homes, medical examiner's offices, and cemeteries the bodies of the recently dead for the purpose of scientific studies without prior consent. The same legal principles, however, do not extend to prehistoric (and sometimes historic) American Indians.

Another facet to consider are court decisions pronouncing "physical mutilation of remains may be expected to distress the next of kin. But where they believe that the treatment will affect the afterlife of the deceased, the impact inevitably is greater" (*Kohn v. the United States* [E.D.N.Y. 1984]). Courts have also ruled that scientific research in itself may constitute this abuse or mutilation (*Hassard v. Lehane* [N.Y. 1911]).

The Nuremberg Code, instituted in 1947 as the result of the amoral scientific experiments conducted by the Nazi regime, established a new standard in ethical medical research, including explicit instructions outlining the requirement of informed consent on behalf of the individual. One of the ten tenets of the code states that "the voluntary consent of the human subject is absolutely essential" in cases involving scientific research, experimentation, and investigation (Mitscherlich and Mielke 1947). The Declaration of Helsinki, which was enacted in 1964, superseding the Nuremberg Code and acting in conjunction with its tenets, dictates twelve basic principles for researchers involved in biomedical research using human subjects (World Medical Organization 1996). The fifth basic principle states, "Every biomedical research project involving human subjects should be preceded by careful assessment of predictable risks in comparison with foreseeable benefits to the subject or to others. Concern for the interests of the subject must always prevail over the interests of science and society."

The National Bioethics Advisory Commission (NBAC) offers policy guidance on ethical issues involved in the use of human biological samples such as human tissue and genetic material, both of which are routinely harvested and utilized in bioarchaeological research.

While neither the Nuremberg Code, the Declaration of Helsinki, nor the NBAC explicitly defines its codes and policy statements as applying to American Indian dead, nor indeed to the bioarchaeological field, a casual inspection of the tenets of each shows that they do not explicitly *exclude* the dead or their families from the need for consent prior to conducting scientific research.

The fact remains that the body of the "dead person is not considered to be a human subject [and these] protections do not apply" but that "it is important to recognize an individual's right to refuse to participate in postmortem research. If the individual has expressed no position before death, the right should be exercisable by his or her next of kin" (Nelkin and Andrews 1998, 271).

Because there is no accepted guidance or policy statement on these matters by the lead American bioarchaeological associations, whether and to what degree the use of dead American Indians is morally acceptable to the osteological researcher now seems to be a matter of personal judgment. This is a nebulous ethical position to assume when dealing in the public arena because it involves research on deceased human beings who have not given their consent, and whose descendants often strongly advocate against using them for these purposes.

2) *Custodial ownership of human remains.* Is it reasonable to assume that cultures in the present can speak for the wishes of their ancestors, and can we presume that the beliefs of the ancient dead are the same as the beliefs of their modern descendants? Should this "cultural uniformatarianism" be applied only toward direct lineal descendants, or can it extend back to pre-historic populations? Who has the moral authority to speak for the remains, and can deceased human beings be considered property, capable of being owned, borrowed, traded, displayed, sold, and experimented upon by other humans and institutions in the absence of consent? In some ways, this is the crux of the debate between bioarchaeologists and American Indians: when the obligation to the dead shifts from a respect for the body of the deceased and the sanctity of his or her grave to respect for the religious or cultural ob-ligations of the living toward their ancestors. Within the anthropological community there often exists a supposition that "as relational bonds become weaker, presumption of custodial claim becomes weaker" (Schrag 2002, 4), a stance not taken by many American Indians, as exemplified by the following quote: "We don't accept any artificial cut-off date set by scientists to separate us from our ancestors. What Europeans want to do with their dead is their business; we have different values" (Walter Echo-Hawk, quoted in Burke Museum Web site, http://www.washington.edu/burkemuseum/kman).

The position that humans may "own" other humans (whether in life or in death) as actual property is one that has obvious parallels in American his-tory, and is not supported either legally or morally. However, the assertion that humans may claim custodial responsibility over the remains of the dead is common. In the case of American Indian remains these claims most often come from two opposing positions: from the descendant Indian populations who are acting as guardians and caretakers of their dead, and from institu-tions such as academic anthropology departments and museums who are in possession of American Indian skeletons.

With respect to the descent populations claiming custodial responsibility for American Indian remains, NAGPRA has placed strict requirements for proving cultural affiliation when dealing with prehistoric remains. While factors such as geographic and temporal continuity, oral history, and lan-guage are factors that can influence the determination of cultural affiliation of ancient American Indian remains, cases like Kennewick Man demonstrate that these criteria are not always enough to prove cultural affiliation to a scientific or legal certainty. When does a human lineage begin and end? Many anthropologists argue that descent is lost in multitudes of human generations, when direct and specific lineages are no longer traceable. This is a weakness in the regulations of NAGPRA and the debate on ancient American skeletal remains: beyond a span of thousands of years, descent is difficult if not impossible to prove. However, NAGPRA simply dictates affiliation can be proven by a "preponderance" of evidence (i.e., more likely than not). Assuming that cultural affiliation is proven between a descendant American Indian population and human remains, does this imply a stronger moral claim to custodial responsibility, or is "the rational connection between an ethnic group and human remains too distant and faint to have any moral standing" (Schrag 2002, 6)?

Museums and academic institutions may also claim custodial responsibility and guardianship for American Indian skeletal remains over competing claims from descendant communities. Essentially, museums are repositories for dead things, with American Indian skeletal remains still occupying many shelves and glass cases even in the post-NAGPRA environment. A common anthropological position regarding ownership of human remains (i.e., Turner 1986) holds that the "remains of the dead belong to the living human race and that museums are, appropriately, the custodians of the remains on behalf of the human race" (Schrag 2002, 3). The interpretation is that museums are adequate and respectful institutions for the housing of both culturally identified and unidentified American Indian human remains, but this viewpoint does not hold a strong moral claim for custodial responsibility when compared to the competing descendant claims asserting cultural affiliation (Handler 1991; Higginbotham 1982).

3) *Intrinsic value of bioarchaeological research.* The scientific community argues that the study of American Indian skeletons benefits all of humanity, especially contemporary Indians by illuminating their past lifeways, adaptations, and histories lost to both time and memory. This is the position bioarchaeologists stress when considering the study and retention of American Indian skeletal remains: "[Anthropologists] . . . believe so strongly in the importance of knowledge and their responsibility to contribute to that knowledge that to not do so would be unthinkable and unethical" (Garza and Powell 2001, 38).

There are legal questions, however, that have to do with the fundamental value of scientific research in scenarios involving the non-consenting dead. Nelkin and Andrews have noted during autopsy protocols that "the law has protected the dead from invasions designed merely to further medical or scientific goals" (1998, 279). This is a point worthy of bioarchaeological consideration: is the research on the non-consenting American Indian dead an appropriate action in cases where the main outcome is to satisfy scientific curiosity (Hamilton 1999)?

Anthropologists maintain that the study and analysis of American Indian cultural and biological remains contribute to scientific advancement and knowledge acquisition, and add to the understanding of those cultures by their modern descendants. Many American Indian groups, however, contend that this stance "cannot be justified on the grounds that the world has a right to this knowledge. Nor can it be justified on the grounds that scientific study provides more reliable or accurate understanding of Native American culture than that embodied in the oral and nonverbal formulations of Native American cultures" (Schrag 2002, 6).

Another concern for American Indians is the use of their dead for the express purpose of promoting research agendas in an attempt to define (or redefine) them as a population and culture. American Indians do not want their own dead used by bioarchaeologists to formulate theories about them. Examples of this type of use of American Indian biological material include the collection in the 1860s of Indian crania ordered by the U.S. surgeon general in order to promote the intellectual inferiority of the American Indian, as well as current anthropological theories situating Kennewick Man as replacing Indian populations as the continent's First Americans.

4) *Prejudicial treatment.* American Indian skeletal remains receive more prejudicial treatment by bioarchaeologists than do the remains of all other ethnic groups. Anthropologists may deny this, or alternately claim that this is a sign of the deep respect they hold for American Indian cultures (Buikstra 1983). Numerous examples exist that demonstrate the uneven treatment of American Indian dead versus equivalent Euro-American dead (Anderson, Zieglowsky, and Shermer 1985; Bieder 1992, 1996; Morton 1848; Nott 1855). Anthropologists must reconcile this fact and determine how to best address this criticism. For example, do the human remains of eighteenth-century Euro-Americans hold less intrinsic biological research value than do the remains of eighteenth-century American Indians? If the answer is no, then anthropologists must reconsider the unequal treatment meted out to American Indians. If the answer is yes, "is it because the research potential is less, or is it because there is a reluctance to do similar research on subjects who share the same ancestry?" ("Scientific Research" 2002, 6). While most bioarchaeologists do not subscribe to this opinion, the veneer of prejudicial

treatment still exists, and bioarchaeologists should address this concern because it remains a divisive issue for modern American Indians.

These legal and moral philosophical arguments may appear abstract when applied toward bioarchaeological research protocols, but they bear consideration as factors inherent in the public perception of anthropological study. Constructive debate on these issues by bioarchaeological researchers would strengthen and clarify the discipline's ethical and scientific positions on the study of American Indian skeletal remains.

## New Beginnings

> We can expect considerable self-consciousness until we relearn what we may never have known, namely, how to let those whose bones we transmute by a strange alchemy into data rest in peace.
> —Grimes 2001, 102

> The Skull Wars, alas, seem far from over. Too many people are still talking past each other. But if archaeologists—of all people—can draw some lessons from the past, perhaps we can rediscover a more human side to our science and come to value once again the importance of face-to-face relationships with those whose ancestors we wish to study.
> —D. Thomas 2000, 276

The increasingly successful utilization of cultural heritage laws like Section 106 of the National Historic Preservation Act and NAGPRA by sovereign American Indian tribes represents a major challenge to the discipline of physical anthropology, increasing by orders of magnitude as more federally recognized tribes form Tribal Historic Preservation Offices and wield growing authority over their own cultural, historical, and biological landscapes.

Many anthropologists have realized that "the very future of anthropological research in North America will be determined primarily by the Tribes rather than by anthropologists" (Deward E. Walker Jr., paraphrased in *Who Owns the Past*), but many biological anthropologists may not be cognizant of the reach and power exerted tribally, publicly, or politically, nor of the subtle shaping of their own disciplines by new tribal imperatives. Within the next few decades, however, bioarchaeologists will be forced to confront these challenges in ways that will unavoidably alter and redefine the discipline as it is practiced in North America (Watkins, Pyburn, and Cressey 2000).

The impression most American Indians maintain concerning bioarchaeologists and their research agendas is largely negative, forged by histories of colonialism and moral neutrality over the collection and study of their dead. Although many tribes such as the Eastern Band of Cherokee Indians are not currently receptive to osteological studies because of cultural and traditional restrictions, other Indian groups are interested in archaeological and bioarchaeological studies of their ancestors. Many examples of tribes and anthropologists collaborating together exist, and include such issues as federal recognition procedures and clarification of tribal land claims (Paredes 1992). In the American West, the Chumash, Zuñi, and Hopi tribes accept and are receptive in many cases to bioarchaeological non-destructive analysis of inadvertently discovered or museum-curated human skeletal remains (E. Adams 1984; Anyon and Ferguson 1995; Anyon and Zunie 1989; Dongoske 1996; Dongoske and Anyon 1997; Walker 2000), while in the Arctic progress among the Inuit has been achieved with the inclusion of indigenous ethnoscience (Bielawski 1992, 1994). Among the Navajo, anthropologists have had a tenuous yet constructive relationship (D. Begay 1991; R. Begay 1997; Klesert 1992; Klesert and Andrews 1988; Klesert and Downer 1990; Martin 1997).

With the authority and enforceability of cultural resource laws, under these new rules of engagement the burden now falls on bioarchaeologists to prove the relevance of their work to others outside academia. American Indian tribal members must be convinced of the value of continuing research on their ancestral dead beyond traditional ontological and epistemological appeals to knowledge and science acquisition.

American bioarchaeology is now facing pressure from external forces to adapt its practices and methodology. Anthropologists labor under a presumption of entitlement when it comes to the study of the dead of North American Indian tribes, and this mantle of science and a responsibility to knowledge are heavy yokes to cast off in light of American Indian appeals to such non-quantifiable factors as religion, morality, ethics, and decency. It is difficult to remember that the very essence of science is an endeavor done by degrees; a slow and steady accumulation of parts when added to the whole gives us that much more insight than we had before. As Walker notes, "When skeletal collections are lost owing to our inability to find equitable solutions that balance the concerns of modern descendants against the need to preserve collections so that future generations will have substantive information about the past, it is perhaps of some solace to remember that we live in an entropic world in which the natural processes of decay and disintegration and the economic and social realities of modern life continuously conspire to destroy the faint traces our ancestors have left for us in the archaeological record" (2000, 31).

Physical anthropologists may react defensively when the moral dimension of their research with American Indian dead is questioned. A necessary response by bioarchaeologists will involve acknowledging the missteps of the past and anticipating the potential for new collaboration with living American Indians. A less constructive tactic to utilize is to label those who question the ethics of studying American Indian skeletal remains as reflective of the agendas of anti-intellectual, anti-science, anti-colonialist, postmodernist, and anti-positivist proponents. This is not a productive approach to employ with legal, political, and public pressure mounting, and it does nothing to elevate the debate within the discipline beyond framing it as a matter of science versus religion, of one academic theory versus another. Bioarchaeological methodology would not be weakened by the inclusion and integration of an ethical component. To the contrary, the addition of a moral dimension would humanize the discipline, make it relevant to living Indian communities, and strengthen its contribution to our understanding of the prehistory of North America.

## Operationalizing Bioarchaeology: Suggestions for Future Praxis

"American archaeology is anthropology or it is nothing," Willey and Phillips (1958, 2) once said, ushering in the new age of processual archaeology. Bioarchaeologists must consider the living as they study the dead, lest they become solely data miners and statistical technicians.

There is a disconnection between the aims of bioarchaeology and the concerns of living American Indians. In the illustration provided in this study via the Eastern Band of Cherokee Indians, there are strong cultural, traditional, and moral prohibitions against contact with, and exposure to, the dead. Physical anthropologists contend that science has a responsibility beyond the Cherokee worldview to the greater public good in studying their human remains, yet anthropological science has in many instances promoted agendas and policies counter to the public interest of American Indians. Bioarchaeologists must depend on their skills as holistic anthropologists to appeal to American Indians who have no obligation to science, do not require that their history be traced through scientific methods, and have not been shown how research on their ancestral dead can prove useful to them.

Practitioners of medical and cultural anthropology have found viable methods of conducting research with the Eastern Band of Cherokee Indians, which enhances the lives of modern Cherokees while contributing to anthropological knowledge. An example of this type of research by Lefler has shown the efficacy of integrating aspects of traditional American Indian culture into modern Eastern Band alcohol rehabilitation and mentoring programs (Lefler 1996, 2001).

Archaeological research on the Qualla Boundary conducted by archaeologist Brett Riggs showcases another applied use of anthropological research that intrigued both the scientific and tribal community. Working with Cherokee potters, Riggs analyzed styles of proto-historic and historic Qualla pottery, which were no longer produced by the Cherokee. This endeavor led to a revitalization in modern Cherokee ceramics manufacture, resulting in the reemergence of the Qualla pottery style among the Cherokee. Bioarchaeologists must also consider similarly applied uses of their research in much the same manner: incorporating dual agendas reflective of both community needs and scholarly interests.

The future of American bioarchaeology can no longer be exclusive of contemporary American Indian involvement. Bioarchaeological method and theory must be reshaped and recast to conform to the new mandates of NAGPRA and cultural resource laws in ways that are sensitive to the needs of American Indians, while at the same time strengthening the discipline's contribution to science and understanding. Academic agendas must now reflect questions that American Indian communities are also interested in posing. Many American Indians argue that they are wholly in possession of their own histories through cultural traditions, religious practices, oral accounts, and memory. They are offended by the implication that it is only through anthropological research that they can know their own past. This backlash toward a Western interpretation of their history also has its roots in the proliferation of negative American Indian stereotypes (Hoxie 1985). Reaction against this lack of a native viewpoint has resulted in a number of novel approaches to native histories, including museums, educational programs, and cultural centers created and run by American Indian tribal groups to promote their own cultures. Bioarchaeologists have an opportunity to contribute to these interpretations, but increasingly, legislative articles like NAGPRA and Section 106 ensure it will be tribes who decide how and to what degree.

The Eastern Band of Cherokee Indians has not been receptive to osteological research as it has thus far been conducted. However, opportunities for bioarchaeological investigation are occasionally presented (e.g., inadvertent discoveries of Cherokee skeletal remains during construction, NAGPRA-mandated inventories of Cherokee-affiliated skeletons in museum collections), and research designs may be developed that interest both the tribe and the bioarchaeologist (Bray 2001; Rodning 2001; Schroedl 1986a, 1986b).

For example, the Cherokee may be interested in the antiquity of their habitation in the region. While the Cherokee themselves are certain of their continuous occupation, there is debate among archaeologists concerning whether the Cherokee are an in situ culture or if they represent a relatively new population migration to the area. If bioarchaeological research can be utilized to show biological and osteological evidence of cultural continuity and long occupation in the region by Cherokee antecedents, this may be of interest to the tribe and could represent a new research avenue for bioarchaeologists to collaboratively and successfully pursue with the Eastern Band of Cherokee Indians.

New guidelines in the training of biological anthropologists must be developed, including the development of ethics statements addressing research with American Indian skeletal remains, additions to graduate physical anthropology curricula focusing on cultural resource legislation, the invitation and participation of tribal members in skeletal biology courses, and the active recruitment of American Indian students to anthropological careers. New avenues for partnerships in bioarchaeological investigations must be identified, including innovative methodologies, non-destructive techniques, synthetic approaches, interdisciplinary collaborations, and cooperative research projects under the aegis of tribal authorities.

The lack of anticipated ethical guidelines for physical anthropologists is detrimental to the discipline, owing to the complex relationship linking American Indians and bioarchaeologists. In the absence of professional and academic incentives to develop and implement ethical human remains policies, graduate training programs in biological anthropology should include instruction on critical issues such as tribal relations, NAGPRA, bioarchaeological ethics, and the impact of cultural resource laws on the discipline. It will be crucial for students to be exposed to the new realities facing them once they become professional biological anthropologists who anticipate working with American Indian skeletal materials.

The forging of collaborative relationships with American Indian communities will be central to the discipline of bioarchaeology in this century. This will require bioarchaeologists to refine their holistic anthropological skills and demonstrate the value of knowledge gained from osteological studies of American Indian remains. One approach to consider is inviting tribal members to lecture to skeletal biology classes. Exposing bioarchaeology students to living American Indians will no doubt lead to increased consideration, deliberation, and potential solutions from all sides of the debate. Another side effect of increased exposure of American Indians to bioarchaeologists may be an increased awareness and understanding of the discipline by tribal communities, as well as a willingness to encourage tribal members to consider careers in anthropology. In order to attract American Indian students, universities and anthropology departments must offer incentives in the form of scholarships, tuition waivers, and internships for Indian students who are interested in pursuing anthropological careers.

These suggestions for adapting the discipline to the post-NAGPRA environment are small steps that can be instituted now. Eventually, new directions for future research and enhanced theoretical frameworks must be created, including tribally initiated research programs and the potential establishment of new scientific paradigms in bioarchaeology with the inclusion of American Indian knowledge, tradition, and guidance. The reality of the situation is summed up by Sockbeson: "Federal laws empower tribes and, for the first time, permit tribes rather than academics to determine the ultimate disposition of Native American human remains. A policy decision has been made by Congress to place tribal social values over the interests of science . . . it is not necessary to balance scientific and public interests in human remains with tribes. Federal law has decided how these interests will be balanced and tribal concerns now outweigh those of the general public and the scientific community" (1994, 158, 160).

The onus is now firmly on American bioarchaeologists to change their methodology and praxis to avoid significant impairment of the discipline. The realities of tribal sovereignty, legal declaration, and public opinion dictate that there simply is no other option.

# 4

# Historical Trauma, Stress, and Diabetes

A Modern Model among the Eastern Band
of Cherokees

*Lisa J. Lefler and Roseanna Belt*

For the Eastern Band of Cherokee Indians (EBCI), the current prevalence of Type 2 or adult-onset diabetes is a pervasive health issue that impacts an overwhelming majority of the community. Tribal members often refer to this disease as "having sugar" (cul sage) or "I'm too sweet" (agee ganast). Some in the community feel that "having sugar" is a direct consequence of a shift from a horticultural/hunting and gathering lifestyle to a "Western" or modern, sedentary lifestyle coupled with a "fast food" culture. Others are beginning to explore the intergenerational and historic impact of assimilation and acculturation. The trauma of boarding schools and removal of people from their land and families has generated stress for generations. Native psychologists like Eduardo Duran and Maria Yellow Horse Brave Heart refer to this effect as "soul wounding." Health professionals and service providers in the Cherokee community are now addressing health and social issues within the context of this historic and intergenerational trauma model. This chapter will share the influence of this model as it is reflected in health care and social services planning and development among the EBCI.

One of the most sobering and pervasive health issues is the rise of diabetes among the EBCI. It is seen as a modern disease, reflecting lifestyle and diet changes during the last one hundred years and particularly during the last two decades. Because these same trends have affected so many indigenous histories, this "modern" disease is also an important issue in the context of global health policy.

A report from the International Diabetes Institute (Zimmet 2001) predicts that by 2010, the number of people in the world with diabetes will double, estimating that over 220 million people will have been diagnosed.

The institute has identified "an urgent need for strategies to prevent this emerging global epidemic of Type 2 diabetes to be implemented. The current situation is a symptom of globalization with respect to its social, cultural, economic and political significance." The report goes on to say this epidemic will not be prevented by Western medical technologies; what is required are "major and dramatic changes in the socio-economic and cultural status of people who are disadvantaged, minority groups, and people in developing nations."

Indigenous peoples have the highest rates of Type 2 diabetes. The Indian Health Service age-adjusted prevalence rate of Type 2 diabetes for American Indians is 69 per 1,000, while the overall U.S. rate is 24.7 per 1,000. According to the National Institute of Diabetes and Digestive and Kidney Disease, about 1 in 8 American Indian adults have diabetes (twice the rate of Caucasians) and deaths due to diabetes are nearly three times higher (November 2002). However, the prevalence of diabetes in adults varies from tribe to tribe, from about 35 percent for those above forty years of age among the Eastern Band of Cherokees in North Carolina, to well over 50 percent among the Pima of Arizona.

On February 8, 2007, the Senate Committee on Indian Affairs listened to just how problematic diabetes is for Indian communities: "In spite of our best efforts and successes so far in treating diabetes, the epidemic of diabetes continues to increase," stated Indian Health Service director Dr. Charles Grim. "Although diabetes is also increasing in the U.S. population as a whole, the increase in the Indian population is far more dramatic. While the prevalence of diabetes in the U.S. population almost doubled between 1980 and 2004, the prevalence of diabetes among American Indians and Alaska Natives was already higher in the early 1980s than in the U.S. population in 2004. Moreover, the prevalence of diabetes among American Indians and Alaska Natives more than doubled during this time period. Indeed, American Indians and Alaska Natives have the highest age-adjusted rates of diabetes (16.3%) among all U.S. racial and ethnic groups and in some communities, the prevalence rate is as high as 60% among adults" (http://indian.senate.gov/public/_files/Grim020807.pdf, pp. 2–3).

Onset of Type 2 diabetes generally occurs during the middle and older years. It is escalating at an alarming rate each year. Even more disconcerting, it is occurring more commonly among younger members of Indian communities; children as young as five among the Havasuapi of northern Arizona (Benyshek 2001) and nine among the EBCI (S. L., personal communication, 2007) have been diagnosed. In the summer of 2002 alone, six EBCI children under the age of fifteen were newly diagnosed. This follows a trend reported by the Naomi Berrie Diabetes Center at Columbia University: "At our institution 30 percent of all our newly diagnosed diabetics under nineteen years of age are Type 2 diabetics. It ranges from 8 to 45 percent of all the new diabetics less than nineteen years old across the country. Texas and California report the most cases. It is shocking, but true" (Vargas, personal communication; Vargas 2002).

Brooke Olson, an anthropologist who works with Native communities to address the problem of diabetes, notes "an alarming increase in diabetes in Indians under the age of 20, and in the past ten years, there has been a two-fold increase in Indian diabetes for those under the age of 16" (2001, 166). A study published in the *American Journal of Public Health* revealed that "from 1990 to 1998, the total number of young American Indians and Alaska Natives with diagnosed diabetes increased by 71%; prevalence increased by 46%" (Acton et al. 2002, 1485). The potential health care cost for greater numbers of Indian youth diagnosed with adult-onset diabetes is daunting for all tribal leaders. By the time a nine- or ten-year-old reaches their twenties or thirties, they are well on their way to the serious diabetes-related health problems that must be addressed and managed, and are facing years of medical visits and costs.

A recent article published in the *American Academy of Pediatrics* emphasizes the growing concern among medical professionals regarding this trend: "Prevention must take highest priority and should focus on decreasing the risk, incidence, and consequences of Type 2 diabetes mellitus among AI/AN children. Primary prevention efforts by primary health care professionals are recommended in two arenas: 1) general community health promotion and health education and 2) clinically based activities" (Gahagan and Silverstein 2003).

An estimated 70 percent of diabetes risk in the United States can be attributed to excess weight (http://www.ncpad.org/disability/fact_sheet. php?sheet=324&view=all&print=yues&PHPSESSID=0). Approximately 85 percent of children diagnosed with Type 2 diabetes are overweight or obese (Urrutia-Rojas and Menchaca 2006). Because prevalence of Type 2 is relatively new among children, true rates have not yet been established, although it is generally agreed that it is increasing at a very steady and steep rate.

Prevention and treatment of diabetes among American Indian communities must be addressed in new ways. Traditional Western approaches to disease causality must have a more indigenous perspective, meaning more holistic. For example, two Cherokee women who work with diabetics on the Qualla Boundary were interviewed by a student intern working with the Cherokee Choices diabetes prevention program. Both of these professionals are involved in a movement that looks at the impact of multigenerational grief and trauma on health and social issues for the tribe. They see lifestyle changes as a result of European contact and assimilation as underlying factors of causality for many health ills such as diabetes. When asked why they thought so many Indians were getting diabetes today they both spoke of lifestyle and culture changes: "Well, we're getting so modern, we no longer need to walk to the store, to visit neighbors, or we no longer have to make a garden 'cause everything is produced right there for us and we have stores that we can just go in and buy whatever we want." The second interviewee said, "Lifestyle change and the foods that we eat, I think that overall way of viewing ourselves in today's society, it's connected to the way we feel about ourselves and I think that the way we feel about ourselves is connected to the choices that we make."

Many others who work with indigenous populations agree that the impact felt by most indigenous peoples is multigenerational. Jennie Joe and Robert Young's edited volume, *Diabetes as a Disease of Civilization,* reflects on the impact of "drastic lifestyle and cultural changes" since World War II. "In addition to the economic, social, and biological consequences of the conquest, there were also undetermined long-term psychological consequences, . . . with a sense of hopelessness and powerlessness, and in most instances, a lifestyle colored by chronic, abject poverty. Unfortunately, despite the passage of time, healing has not occurred" (1994, 7).

The assimilation process has fostered, in their words, "problems such as alcoholism, suicide, homicide, low self-esteem, and the emergence of 'new' health problems such as hypertension, cancer, and diabetes" (1994, 6). Eduardo Duran also underscores the impact of colonialism on Native communities and identifies many social and health ills as an intergenerational transfer of post-traumatic stress. He states, "the lack of awareness of the historical legacy limits true understanding of American Indian health status and fosters the practice of blaming Indian people for alcohol-related and other health-related morbidity" (1998, 347).

Waldram, Herring, and Young (1995), Sellers (2000), and Feuer's (2001) diabetes research among Canada's First Nations communities speak to similar issues. All see the rise in prevalence of Type 2 as part of modernization or Westernization of their communities as more traditional ways of life are diminished. Cherokee studies colleague Jenny James characterizes the trauma of assimilation and disruption of traditional culture on Cherokee health as a move from a "harmony ethic" to a "Western stress ethic" (personal communication, November 2002). Loomis and Wing (1990), Pearce (1996), and McMichael (1999) all urge a shift from reductionist, individual-centered studies of disease causation to ones that operate at a population-level and consider larger, contextual influences on health. Marmot and Wilkinson's volume *Social Determinants of Health* provides "good evidence" that history, life experiences, and stressors trigger physiological responses that lay the groundwork for and/or exacerbate diseases including diabetes (2001, 26).

These considerations are applicable to the EBCI. As much of the ethnographic and historic literature relays, a rapid era of change impacted the traditional subsistence strategies and lifestyle of the Cherokee. Records left by Timberlake (1765), Bartram (1791), Butrick/Payne (n.d. but recorded volumes in early nineteenth century), and others indicate extreme proficiency at using the vast natural resources of the southern Appalachian region. A plethora of edible wild plants, domesticated plants, fish, fowl, and wild meats provided a varied and healthy diet. Goodwin's analysis of diet concluded that the "farming base was so strong, a single acre in mixed planting could provide enough food for one person per year" (1977, 55). But as McLoughlin (1986), points out, by the mid-1700s the pressures of contact and integration into a Euro-American economy fueled exploitation of resources and loss of land and resource holdings. Ensuing wars led to devastation of crops, towns, and a traditional way of life. During the scourge of the late eighteenth century, Grant's troops were ordered to "pull up beans, peas, corn and demolish every eatable thing in the country" (Goodwin 1977, 104). For the Cherokees left after forced removal in 1838, discrimination and trauma left an indelible mark. Missionaries devalued Cherokee beliefs and spirituality, and federal authorities began a legacy of Indian policies that were intent on assimilation and "whitening" the Cherokee way of life.

Indian agents, referred to in a less paternal way as "superintendents" of Cherokee boarding schools, provided annual reports to the Bureau of Indian Affairs. Through these narratives from 1910 to 1918, we catch a glimpse of how drastically Cherokee subsistence and diet has since changed. One dated June 29, 1910, describes the climate of the Qualla Boundary.

It is particularly favorable for plant growth, and is well adapted for agriculture and horticulture. In ordinary seasons, the fruit is superior both in quality and quantity to that in most sections [of western North Carolina]. It is estimated that about 90 percent of the EBCI earn their living by tilling the soil, the average number of acres cultivated by heads of families being about 30, including the portion used for pasture. . . . The main crop of the Indians of this reservation is corn, but a considerable quantity of other grains and vegetables such as beans, potatoes, oats, etc. are produced. The live stock industry is carried on in connection with regular farming work.

The estimated 800 head of cattle and oxen, 200 horses, 800 pigs, and 400 sheep were, in his words, "well distributed among the Indians." At this time, the superintendent recorded the Cherokee population to be around 2,000 enrolled members occupying about 63,000 acres, much of which wasn't suitable for agricultural purposes (although later he reported that about 12,000 acres were being cultivated).

In the 1914 report, it was noted that almost all families had a garden with the principal crops of corn, beans, potatoes, wheat oats, and grass. The main staple of their diet was corn in the form of cornbread and lye hominy, beans, and salt pork. Although almost every family kept a cow, milk and butter weren't commonly used by everyone, nor were beef and mutton preferred meats. Often pigs were turned out "wild" to roam freely, but they were enticed to stay close to home by feedings where they would come down the mountains to periodically access this additional food source. Wild turkeys were enticed the same way and were an added source of protein.

Recent ethnographic research by Heidi Altman (2006) suggests fish, namely trout, were also an important food among the EBCI. Fishing was a family activity, and as Altman's research shows, it was an important and integral part of Cherokee subsistence. Families also raised chickens and some kept bees for honey. Eggs and honey were a source of revenue, as were surplus vegetables and fruit such as apples and strawberries. The caption to a photograph showing one family with their bees read, "his output of honey during the last year was over 2,000 pounds." The 1915 report mentioned that the agricultural exhibit, the first attempt made by farmers from Cherokee, was better than at neighboring county fairs.

In contrast, today only 1 percent, or 150 acres, of land formerly used are cultivated on the Boundary. The local farm service agent estimated that only 40–50 home gardens were still grown, mainly in Big Cove, Soco, and Birdtown, with the average size being two-tenths of an acre or less. He said that about 10 acres of tomatoes were leased to non-tribal members, and about 40 acres of corn were grown. Of that all but six acres were cultivated for livestock feed, the rest for Indian corn flour, which is sold to tourists. He added that virtually no one kept bees any longer and that most everyone gets their food from the grocery store or some other commercial venue (personal communication, November 2002).

Similarly, use of the tribal cannery remains slim. The individual who oversees this operation shared that over 60 percent of those who use this service are above the age of sixty, with no requests from those under the age of about forty. The majority who do use the cannery purchase their produce (personal communication, November 2002).

The use of home gardens has been in steady decline since the 1930s. A shift in the economic base of the Cherokees began with the handicraft revival, the opening of the Great Smoky Mountain National Park, and incoming mountain visitors who brought tourist dollars and demand for baskets and other Cherokee crafts. By the mid-1900s, the decline in subsistence farming was noticeable. One of Ray Fogelson's (1958) informants from the Big Cove community during the late 1950s commented, "You know, when I was a girl this whole bottom was covered with corn and beans, and people had hogs. We had all we wanted to eat. The man that raised me had about thirty hogs. (My mother gave me away.) He said that when he died, it would all go away and it did, too. People don't farm anymore—rather work for cash, I guess—but things were better then" (quoted in Kupferer 1966).

There was also a shift in health during this period. Health during the first two decades of the twentieth century was reported to be generally good. Notable ills were whooping cough, hookworms, and an occasional case of diphtheria or chickenpox. Most of the health concerns were related to poor sanitation conditions around the homes. Photos within these reports through 1918 show families in and around their homes, schoolchildren, men playing stickball, and folks attending other events (e.g., the Indian Fair), all with few to no signs of obesity. Some from the community have commented that people walked much, much more than they do today. Several have stated that folks walked an average seven miles a day, estimating how far it was for people to walk to and from community stores, schools, and workplaces.

In contrast, health concerns today include metabolic disorders, with diabetes as a major focus. Even though symptoms of diabetes or "having sugar" may have existed before the 1950s, the disease was not identified nor understood in the community until the early 1960s. Frank Starr, under the direction of Franz Boas, collected stature measurements and genealogical information on 459 Eastern Cherokees in 1892. Deann Stivers's work traced 32 percent of the descendants from Starr's study and showed that stature had increased, particularly among females. But there was a "tendency among older individuals to gain adipose tissue in the trunk region" (1990, 109). She also notes that although diabetes was not listed as being treated, the presence of chronic sores and the extended treatment time needed were indications of difficulty in healing, a common symptom of diabetes. She states, "Older Eastern Cherokees can identify the presence of symptoms of diabetes at least since the early 1920s" (108).

Pat Quiggins's work (1990) also surveys the issue of diabetes among the EBCI. She cites that incidence of diabetes was concentrated in individuals aged forty-five to sixty-four. Her study, compared with the first recorded study of diabetes among the EBCI by Stein et al. (1965), shows a steady increase in the prevalence of diabetes from 17.2 percent to 25 percent in 1988. The numbers have now increased to 35 percent, including younger and younger cases of adult onset. Rhonda Terry's research in a more remote community of the EBCI shows that "in the Snowbird Township, clinic staff estimate approximately 50 percent of the adults have diabetes" (1982, 2). This was up from 24 percent in 1975. At that time, one of three main factors that contributed to the risk of developing diabetes was advancing age. Today, with an increase in diagnoses of adult-onset diabetes in youth under the age of fifteen, childhood obesity is a related factor. The percentage of EBCI children who are overweight or obese is significantly higher than the national average. One may project from this factor that diabetes will be on the rise among the EBCI over the next twenty years unless serious prevention measures are implemented. EBCI medical director Ann Bullock refers to the projected numbers related to future health care issues and expenditures of diabetes care as a "tsunami effect." Tribal members are being diagnosed earlier and living longer, which means long-term health care expenditures. These are serious issues that affect almost all tribes in the United States and are a top priority and concern. The EBCI are taking a proactive approach and conducting monthly diabetes committee meetings including health care providers, representatives of multiple tribal agencies, and community members to plan and implement preventive and intervention initiatives.

Turning to preventive measures, a 1990 national survey of almost 9,500 Native American school-aged children showed that "overweight prevalence was high for all ages and for both sexes" (Broussard et al. 1995, 290S). Obesity has been understood as one of the predictors of diabetes and has been associated with depression in adolescents (Goodman and Whitaker 2002). Current literature concerning diabetes indicates a milieu inclusive of depression, stress, and obesity. More studies are providing plausible explanations of their links (see Sapolsky 1998; Bullock 2001b; Hjemdahl 2002; and Brunner et al. 2002). These issues combined demonstrate a need for study of young diabetics and the factors that influence their health. Mary Story (1980) conducted a study of food and nutrient intake practices among Cherokee high school students in the late 1970s. Her observations included a high level of obesity among eighth, ninth, and tenth grade students. She recommended that more nutrition and "weight awareness" information needed to be included in the elementary school curriculum "since many students in Cherokee were already obese in the eighth grade" (100).

Because diet is such an important part of understanding childhood obesity, the Cherokee Choices program conducted surveys among fifth graders that included questions regarding food choices and frequencies, as well as activity schedules and health behavior. For example, the results of a questionnaire among Cherokee fifth graders show that on average, children eat at local fast food establishments about twice a week, and about 18 percent of the sample (n = 82) eat there three or more times a week, with a majority eating out about five times a week. Sixty-five percent of the children said they watched television and/or movies "a lot," while 52 percent said they played video games "a lot." One must consider that these changes in diet and lifestyle also reflect the use of technology (cars, television, computers), which makes it possible for people to live without "community" and further slide into the paradigm of Western individualism.

Sallie Arch, a diabetic and elder of the tribe, writes, "This disease has affected most of the enrolled members here on the Cherokee Reservation mainly due to the changes of our lifestyle and not eating healthy foods such as our traditional foods that we gather every season. This is happening at a fast pace. Today, my heart is heavy with emotions from the cries of my people who are asking a question, 'why?'" (2002).

There has been a line drawn between the shift from a farming-based economy to a tourist-based economy and the change in diet and level of physical activity. These changes have contributed to those factors, which increase obesity and subsequent risk for Type 2 diabetes. Of urgent concern are the implications of these lifestyle and diet changes ensconced in a tourist/casino-driven economy, and the simultaneous need to develop a viable diabetes prevention program that seeks to reduce obesity, inspire increased physical activity, and improve nutrition. One of the cultural identifiers that may be an asset to such a program is the call to revitalization, community activity, and involvement. After a discussion about these issues, one community leader called on tribal council members to attend a community dinner and visit with their elders. She also hopes to revitalize community by bringing back "shoebox dinners" that, as she put it, "will encourage people to visit with one another again." A shoebox dinner is "Indian food" prepared and bought and/or taken in a shoebox to an elder in the community. One then is expected to have dinner and spend time with that elder. Proceeds may go to a community center or some other fund-raising event.

As the literature shows, "gains in material consumption and technology do not ensure gains in health" (McMichael 1999). Gro Harlem Brundtland, director general of the World Health Organization (the "E. F. Hutton" of health policy and globalization), said on World Health Day in 2002, "the world is experiencing a rapidly spreading epidemic of inactivity, poor diet and increased tobacco use" (WHO 2002). The message was a call to action for global policymakers to help individuals make positive lifestyle change.

The case of the EBCI adds to the chorus of global voices calling for healthy lifestyles for all peoples, their environment, and future generations. Olson's research concerning diabetes among Native populations understood that "historical and epidemiological perspectives are essential in understanding the complex causal factors associated with diabetes and how to minimize these factors in education and treatment programs." She adds, "One significant factor that needs to be highlighted is the role of acculturation, or the processes whereby major culture changes are forced onto a society as a consequence of intensive firsthand contact or conquest" (2001, 165).

Considering the enormity of diabetes as a major health concern, the EBCI are proactively responding to this endemic health issue via their health providers and a group of concerned community members who are taking a new look at causality and intervention. The emerging perspective on the intersection between diabetes, stress, and the impact of the traumatic history of the EBCI is being talked about within the community and among health providers. These folks assert that modern medicine is finally catching up with the understanding of Indian people: stress, poverty, and trauma can make you sick. Now, it may even make you "have sugar."

When we think of Western medicine, we usually think of new technology and empirically trained "elite" professionals who see individuals for illnesses and typically view disease from a reductionist perspective. Helman describes the basic underpinnings of modern medicine as "scientific rationality; emphasis on objective, numerical measurement; emphasis on physiochemical data; mind-body dualism; the view of diseases as entities; and an emphasis on the individual patient, rather than on the family or community" (1994, 86–87).

More traditional perspectives of health among the Cherokee could be described as holistic and pervasive. Everything is culturally tied into health, including stickball preparation and play, ceremonies, relationships with plants and animals, diet, dances, songs, and taboo violations. One member of the community whose father practiced medicine until his death in the early 1980s gave this analogy: "Sickness is an entity that can come and visit. It is a natural part of the world and a balance has to be created between them. For example, we live with a lot of bears, but don't let them live in your house. You must keep them at bay. It is a rational existence; one that you can deal with, if you just avoid visits and long stays by sickness. It was the medicine man's job to figure out what was in its suitcase and how to bring back the balance in the 'tired' one's relationships" (Lefler's field notes, Cherokee, NC, September 11, 2003).

One of the ways traditional and Western practitioners differ is in their approach to the patient. A Western doctor will ask a patient to identify physical symptoms that must be observable and measurable to be validated as medical. If this cannot be done, the problem is assumed to be psychosomatic. A traditional practitioner is more likely to take a subjective approach and seek an in-depth history of how a person has been living. My aforementioned consultant remembered his father not asking someone what was wrong physically or symptomatically when a person came to see him. Instead he asked other questions to figure out what had happened to the individual over a period of time. This represents a more holistic and emic approach to health care.

When a Native diabetes clinician was asked how physicians should be addressing illnesses such as diabetes, she responded by saying, "Today we have the opportunity to address these critical issues by recognizing how the feelings connected to losses [relating to our culture] affect our physical, mental, and emotional health. It is very clear that when we start talking about the experiences of our ancestors, we can feel within our own bodies the pain of what happened many years ago as though we were there" (Lefler's field notes, Cherokee, NC, August 2002).

Her response is referred to by many as multigenerational or historic grief and trauma and has growing significance for health providers in many ethnic populations, particularly American Indians. "For the past three centuries, extensive and sometimes forcible sociocultural changes have impacted on the lifestyle and culture of Native Americans. Each cycle of experience with non-Indians in each historical period has left an imprint on the health picture of American Indians" (Joe and Young 1993, 5). This quote appears under the heading "Diabetes and Cultural Change: The Price of Civilization" in *Diabetes as a Disease of Civilization*. The premise of this text is that diabetes is a modern disease brought on by the encroachment of Western values and ideals.

There is no doubt that European invasion brought indigenous people swift biological, economic, social, and psychological change. Eduardo Duran, a native psychologist and coauthor with Bonnie Duran of *Native American Postcolonial Psychology* (1995), identifies the social and medical manifestations of this pervasive change as a "soul wound" and feels this concept has been known in Indian country for many generations. As the term implies, the trauma seen, felt, and heard is transformed deep within the psyche and erupts into forms of abusive, anxious, and depressive behaviors resulting from generations of exploitation, assimilation, and marginalization. Duran underscores the impact of colonialism as an intergenerational transfer of post-traumatic stress. The cyclic and connecting web of tragic and often confusing events leads to adaptation and restructuring of the world around them, often with what a local Cherokee counselor identifies as "psychic numbing" or desensitization of the trauma they incur.

Intergenerational or historical grief and trauma is a model many are using to explain the causality for physical and social ills that are pervasive in Indian country. Maria Yellow Horse Brave Heart of the Takini Network defines this model as "a cumulative and psychic wounding across generations related to massive root trauma" (Duran 2005). Much like the notion of soul wound, Manson et al. also refer to this concept as "wounded spirit" (1998), a term most Native Americans quickly identify as a phenomenon that manifests in substance abuse, suicide, domestic violence, post-traumatic stress disorder and a host of other social and physical ills.

While stresses associated with the overarching umbrellas of assimilation and acculturation are ongoing, stress is part of the day-to-day routine of survival and adaptation and is manifested in health problems such as diabetes, cardiovascular disease, metabolic disorders, and depression. The following passage comes from Jerome Kroll's editorial in a recent volume of the *Journal of the American Medical Association* dedicated to the complex issues relating to such trauma.

> Although final common pathways are inevitably mediated biologically (neuroendocrine functional alterations) and psychologically (the trio of re-experiencing, avoidance, and arousal), the long-term consequences of trauma are far-reaching. The context in which the trauma

occurs, the age and stage of life of the traumatized person, the associated losses of family and cultural coherence, characteristics of the person prior to the trauma, the conditions of life after the traumatic encounter, and the symbolic and moral meanings attached to the traumatic events all affect the expression and experience of posttraumatic stress responses. (2003, 669)

Ann Bullock, M.D., has been addressing a variety of health and academic audiences, connecting trauma and stress to one of the most endemic health issues in Indian country, Type 2 diabetes. Her message echoes the works of Sapolsky (1998, 2003), McEwen (2002), van der Kolk and Fisler (1994), and Kroll (2003), detailing the physiological responses to stress. Bullock describes the connection: "Stress and trauma have direct effects on diabetes risk through the Hypothalamic-Pituitary-Adrenal (HPA) Axis and the Autonomic Nervous System. If stress and trauma, both past and present, lead to insulin resistance through neuroendocrine and behavioral/coping mechanisms, there is little wonder there is a diabetes epidemic surging through Indian country. After her work among the Navajo, Kathleen Huttlinger also concludes, 'diabetes needs to be considered a manifestation of intergenerational PTSD'" (Bullock 2001a).

In citing the work of Wamala et al. (1999) and recent articles from the *Journal of the American Medical Association,* Bullock shows the connection between environmental stress and the physiological impact of putting those original "fight or flight" responses on tilt, thus clearing the way for metabolic disasters. Also included in her talks are slides with figures and multiple schemas of the brain, neural pathways, hormonal responses, and input of stimuli from outside agents depicting the cause-and-effect mechanisms that are blueprints for diseases like diabetes.

Bullock is also a member of a local organization made up of concerned medical and tribal people among the EBCI, the Tsalagi Aniyvwiya Dinisdelisgi (Cherokee Indian Helpers), who are developing a model for community-wide intervention and education concerning the impact of historical grief and trauma on the mental, physical, and spiritual health of their people. This organization has been involved in activities to promote the use of the historical grief and trauma paradigm in tribal agency services. This movement, though in its initial stages, is generating dialogue about a painful and difficult past and initiating a vision of healing and a hopeful future.

One of the group's founding members, Patty Grant, recently received the

Peacemaker's Award from the Western North Carolina Mediation Services for her efforts in providing historical grief and trauma education in the region. She has been involved in workshops not only on the Qualla Boundary but also nationally. She has also been working with a Catholic liaison and conducting workshops with Catholic churches within a hundred-mile radius of Cherokee. Targeting church involvement came early in the organization's development. Committee members felt that a good way to begin the education process in the community was to involve local churches. To kick off an introduction of this topic into local congregations a "Healing and Reconciliation Day" took place in Cherokee. A variety of ministers and church representatives took part in the daylong event, allowing those attending to hear public apologies from area church leaders. Announcing this event, the local paper said that "various churches will ask forgiveness from Cherokee and other Native Americans for failing to recognize their sacred worth by misrepresenting the message of Jesus Christ" ("Cherokee Healing" 2002). For some denominations, this was a valued opportunity to express their apologies. The local Methodist minister acknowledged that "the church must atone for its sins before it can minister to the Cherokee." He continued by saying, "From my perspective as a white male, I see a need for the white church to apologize for the oppression by Christian missionaries of Native American people; we thought we had to Europeanize them to evangelize. I am not apologizing for the Gospel. But I do apologize for how we perverted the Gospel in the name of Jesus and oppressed God's people" (Quintin and Ostendorff 2002).

However, one Baptist minister interviewed by a local reporter dismissed the event, saying, "As far as I'm concerned, it's a waste of time, there's nothing to apologize for" (Quintin and Ostendorff 2002). Noted Cherokee historian John Finger agreed, stating, "The Cherokee largely welcomed missionaries into their culture, though not initially for religious purposes. They recognized the value of being taught to read and write in English." He concluded his interview: "I think it has been a relatively happy marriage for more than a hundred years. I'm sort of bemused these churches are offering a formal apology. I wasn't aware there was any particular problem" (Quintin and Ostendorff 2002).

When asked, the former chief agreed an apology wasn't necessary: "Personally I think the past is history and I don't hold present-day people responsible. All we can do is live today's life and do the best we can today" (Quintin and Ostendorff 2002). However, a few months later in a speech to tribal members, Chief Jones said,

I suspect that people outside the Tribe and Reservation do not understand our wounds. But they are deep and ancient. In spite of millions
of dollars pouring into Cherokee, we cannot let go of the past. We cannot forget that time and time again Cherokee people have been dis-
appointed, have been lied to, have been taken advantage of. No matter
how many generations will pass, we will never forget the removal, the
loss of our lands and our way of life. We cannot forget the way we were
made strangers in our own land. We cannot forget the Tribe has had
to fight for its very existence over and over again, just to protect our
lands from being taken away from us once more. We cannot forget the
dependency that was forced upon us through the government schools,
through BIA restrictions, or the isolation from non-Cherokee people
during the years when we were denied rights available to others because we were Indians. (Jones 2003)

Patty Grant, a primary presenter of the trauma model and an enrolled
EBCI member, stated, "The soul wounds that were inflicted on our ancestors generations ago continue to affect us in many ways emotionally, physically, mentally, and spiritually. We as a community need to begin the healing
process by acknowledging the pain inflicted by European culture through
forced assimilation and colonization. In order to begin this process we must
start by openly addressing these issues and allow the healing to begin." De-
scribing her attempts to share this message, she said, "Initially people have
a mixed feeling. The topic presents a certain amount of curiosity for those
Indians that can identify fully with parents or grandparents that went to
boarding school. It triggers all kinds of emotions. But for those who can't
relate, they are just much more removed from the cultural aspects of being
Cherokee" ("Cherokee Healing" 2002).

She shared one of the most powerful experiences she had after presenting at one of the community centers in Cherokee: "Don't you remember
when——followed us out of the Painttown meeting? She said for the first
time she understood why her mother, a boarding school survivor, had acted
and treated her and her siblings the way she did for all those years. She finally understood the pain of her mother's losses that she passed down to her
children. She had become numb and couldn't touch us and couldn't tell us
that she loved us" (Lefler's field notes, Cherokee, NC, 2003).

Another community member, a twenty-seven-year-old mother of one,
shared how she felt about the presentations and billboards that were reflecting messages of historical trauma.

The idea of intergenerational trauma and grief is a concept new to the Cherokees. We know that the history of the Cherokee people has had negative effects on those that suffered the abuse. There are many people who feel disconnected and don't have a sense of belonging because of the loss of the cultural influence and tradition in the home. I have often wondered how I could deal with the feelings and emotions I have inside of me. I didn't personally experience all of these things, but I feel the pain and anger and sorrow and bitterness from these events and I don't know what to do with them. How do I handle this? How do any of us handle this? (Lefler's field notes, Cherokee, NC, August 2003)

After the discussions of how continuing the cycle of a self-destructive lifestyle stems from intergenerational grief, the message is one of how to restore the balance in one's life and heal with dignity. This modern movement provides a reconnection to the values and traditions of what is Cherokee. It involves people actively changing their ideas and beliefs about themselves (e.g., the fatalism of being Cherokee and dying on dialysis, as one fifty-two-year-old woman related) and making behavior changes in diet and lifestyle. A new health challenge program initiated by the EBCI's Health and Medical Division, Cherokee Choices brings nutritionists to tribal worksites and promotes nutritional education, increased physical activity, and methods of stress reduction. This model program has shown initial success in weight loss and reduction of body fat by participants. Cherokee Choices, a Centers for Disease Control and Prevention–funded program, also provides mentoring to promote wellness in the local elementary school. This project works with children in the Cherokee school and has shown positive results in children's self-reports of dealing with stressful events in their lives.

As recent studies have shown, dealing with issues of adverse childhood experiences (ACE) is imperative for healthy adulthood. ACEs are considered a critical predictor of a variety of behaviors and chronic diseases including heart disease, illicit drug use, smoking, alcoholism, depression, sexual promiscuity, and other issues (Anda et al. 1999, 2002; Dube et al. 2003; Dong et al. 2004; Koss 2005). The intersection of genetics and environment is becoming more prominent in the medical literature. A clearer picture is emerging concerning the interconnectedness of mind and body and the impact of environment and history on the health of an individual and a population. Duran cautions us to keep in mind regarding Indian clients, "Native people don't exist separately from the energy and spirit of their people, they are a collective and living history" (2002, 9). Resiliency *is* modernity for Cherokee people.

The endemic problem of diabetes among American Indian people requires the help of both traditionalists and Western-trained health professionals in finding a solution. Several factors of causality—high-fat diet, sedentary lifestyle, being genetically "front-end loaded," stress/historical trauma, as well as new research into fetal origins—are all part of the equation. Bruce D. Perry and Maia Szalavitz's work (2006), as well as that of Shonkoff and Phillips with the National Research Council and the Institute of Medicine (2000), show what happens to children who are deeply impacted by severe stress and trauma. They conclude that exposure to trauma and neglect, even in the earliest months and years of life, can shape the brain and set the stage for health issues as adults. We know environment and culture are important in fostering healthy childhood and adult development. Health directors in Cherokee are very interested in the approach of providing services with the full life cycle in mind. In reviewing recent literature regarding historical trauma, soul wounding, stress, and chronic disease, they also believe that the foundation for general wellness and health is formed very early in life. For this reason they are working on providing more focused care with their expectant mothers, infants, toddlers, young children and their parents, and caregivers. Our larger society focuses largely on providing services for older children and investing in them particularly when they come of age, attend college, and enter young adulthood. The approach the EBCI are taking reflects special services and investment in the very young.

For example, a language immersion program places children in a Cherokee-speaking-only classroom at the tribal day care. Those who have participated in the program consistently comment on the improved self-esteem and confidence of the children. A full-time registered nurse is stationed at the tribal day care where she can attend to the children's medical needs and discuss diet and other health issues with family members. A plan is being developed to assign a nurse to expectant mothers so that she may help care for the mother and new child for a prolonged period of time, providing vaccinations and other medical services and guidance. There are nurses and licensed counselors assigned to the elementary and high schools as well as a full staff at the Cherokee youth center that provides health and mental health services to children and adolescents. Parenting programs are available through the tribe's Health and Medical Division for assistance with issues ranging from smoking cessation and weight management to multiple diagnoses of health and mental health issues.

All of these programs are being developed or already in existence because the EBCI are trying to provide services for the whole person throughout the life cycle. It is a socialized health system that is being tailored to meet the needs of a people who have been living in a system of colonization for more than five hundred years. There are also plans for elders and traditional healers to talk about wellness and health issues while Western-trained medical staff listen and learn about how culture plays a central part in how they address patients and their health problems. It is hoped that new ways can be found to establish more culturally appropriate medical services with a relationship between patient and healer that is didactic for both. "We are in the living and healing process together," one elder shared. "Our conjurors would engage us in a dialogue about our lives and relationships with all other things, and then join with us in a process whereby we could become well and in balance again. You wouldn't just sit in a room and get talked to and were asked to take pills and when you came back and weren't well, get written up for non-compliance" (Lefler's field notes, Cherokee, NC, August 2003).

# 5
# The Effect of Traditional Dietary Practices on Contemporary Diseases among the Eastern Band of Cherokee Indians

*David N. Cozzo*

The Eastern Band of Cherokee Indians are descendants of the original Cherokee Nation, a group that once controlled a large region of the southeastern United States including southern Virginia and West Virginia, northern Georgia, South Carolina, Alabama, western North Carolina, eastern Tennessee, and most of Kentucky. After the forced removal of Native Americans from the eastern United States in 1838, most of the Cherokee were relocated to the Indian Territory in Oklahoma. But approximately 1,000 remained in the mountainous region of North Carolina; some became citizens of the state and others eluded federal troops in the isolated terrain. According to the official tribal Web site (http://www.nc-cherokee.com/), there are currently more than 13,400 enrolled tribal members. The 2000 census found 8,092 members residing on the 56,621-acre Qualla Boundary, tribal land that is held in trust by the federal government.

The process of acculturation among the Cherokee began well before the removal, but the pace has quickened over the last century. Before removal there were essentially two factions among the Cherokee. In the southern end of their territory below the Snowbird Mountain range in southwestern North Carolina, the progressive faction had adopted many of the traits of their white neighbors. Many of these progressive Cherokees were of mixed Indian/white heritage and had adopted Euro-American lifestyles to demonstrate their level of "civilization" to their white neighbors. The conservative faction was predominantly composed of full-blood Cherokees who lived in relative isolation in the higher region of the southern Appalachian Mountains. The land in this area was considered of little value, having few mineral resources and little fertile bottomland, and there was little incentive to enforce the removal decree (Neely 1979, 156).

Changes throughout the twentieth century hastened the rate of acculturation. Formal education was introduced to the Cherokee in 1880 by the Quakers, but twelve years later the schools were taken over by the Bureau of Indian Affairs (BIA). The conditions in the BIA schools were exceedingly harsh and students were often sent far from the reservation and punished for speaking Cherokee. Economic trends were also a factor. The population on the reservation increased while the land area remained the same. The Cherokee farms were small and had little tillable acreage. By the 1950s, only 10 percent of Cherokee families obtained their livelihood by farming and by the 1970s the number of families sustained by farm income was negligible. Most income was from wage labor positions off the reservation or from the tourism industry, but this was inadequate to meet the needs of most households (Neely 1979, 168). Living conditions for the Cherokee mirrored those of other reservation situations across the United States; the population had outgrown the resources of marginal land and inadequate sources of outside employment.

Many of the health problems attributed to the Cherokee, and most Native American groups as well, can be directly attributed to poverty, a sedentary lifestyle, and the loss of traditional dietary patterns. Poverty is known to affect food choices and accompanied nutritional status, which can lead to the development of chronic diseases. This is especially true in low-income, rural areas where access to healthful foods is restricted by small markets carrying few fresh foods and by limited food budgets (Stroehla, Malcoe, and Velie 2005). While the poverty rate for most groups dropped in 1989, only the rate for Native Americans increased to 27 percent, compared with 10 percent for the entire U.S. population (Trosper 1996). The loss of high-activity subsistence patterns such as hunting, farming, and gathering wild foods led to a more sedentary lifestyle and an associated rise in the occurrence of obesity (Narayan 1996). Traditional diets that were low in saturated fat, high in fiber, high in complex carbohydrates, and adequate in high-quality protein sources were replaced with overly refined, high-carbohydrate, high-fat, low-fiber diets (Stroehla, Malcoe, and Velie 2005; Wiedman 1989). By the mid-1980s, many Cherokee youths were unfamiliar with their traditional foods and appeared to be losing that connection to their heritage (Story, Bass, and Wakefield 1985).

Obesity due to the loss of traditional diets and activity patterns is becoming less a result of poverty in Cherokee and more a reflection of a pervasive national trend. The introduction of gaming to the Cherokee community has raised the standard of living substantially. Associated with the new affluence is the proliferation of fast food restaurants, which in the past primarily served the tourist industry but are now heavily relied upon by the larger community. The increased reliance on fast food, with an associated rise in the consumption of sugar-sweetened beverages, is a prominent factor in national obesity rates (St.-Onge, Keller, and Heymsfield 2003; Moreno and Rodríguez 2007). For young people, these rates are exacerbated by long hours spent watching television and playing video games (Hanley et al. 2000).

In this essay I will consider three chronic diseases known or suspected to be a problem among the Eastern Cherokee and view them in light of traditional Cherokee dietary practices. The three diseases under consideration are diabetes mellitus, gallstones, and cervical cancer. Diabetes is known to be a serious problem among the Cherokee, but there is strong evidence that it can be managed through diet and exercise. The prevalence of gallstones among the Cherokee is not available in the literature on Native American health issues, but they are known to be a serious problem in Native Americans in general and are closely associated with obesity and diabetes. The Cherokee have a very high prevalence of both and are very likely to have a high rate of gallbladder disease. Cervical cancer was, until recently, a very serious problem for Cherokee women. Rates are now to those of the general U.S. population, but the close association with cervical cancer and diet suggests that improved dietary status would reduce these rates even further.

The traditional Cherokee diet may be difficult to define. Archaeological evidence suggests that the region of the southern Appalachian Mountains has been continuously occupied for over ten thousand years (Chapman et al. 1982). Subsistence strategies ranged from hunter-gatherers to gardeners to agriculturists (Yarnell and Black 1985). Introduced species were quickly assimilated and became important components of the Cherokee diet (Goodwin 1977). For the purposes of this chapter, the traditional Cherokee diet will consist of crops that were grown at the time of European contact and have remained important contributions to Cherokee subsistence, crops introduced by Europeans and adopted by the Cherokee from the fifteenth through the late nineteenth centuries, and wild foods reported to be used by the Cherokee. Deleterious additions or changes to the diet will also be noted.

The arrangement of the chapter is as follows: a description of diabetes mellitus, gallstones, and cervical cancer that includes their significance to the general Native American population, the known or suspected etiology of each disease, complications associated with each condition, and aspects of the disease relevant to the Cherokee. This is followed by a more in-depth explanation of acculturation among the Cherokee and an analysis of the traditional diet as it pertains to each of the diseases.

## Diabetes

Diabetes mellitus is a chronic condition affecting carbohydrate metabolism. The most conspicuous symptom is elevated glucose levels in blood and urine due to inadequate production or utilization of insulin. Other symptoms include the production and excretion of copious amounts of urine, excessive thirst, and an increase in appetite. In advanced cases the circulatory system is impaired and there is weight loss and weakness. Untreated diabetes leads to nausea, headache, delirium, labored breathing due to insufficient oxygen uptake, and eventually coma or death (C. Thomas 1997, 527).

Diabetes is classified into two syndromes: Type 1, or insulin-dependent diabetes mellitus (IDDM), and Type 2, or non-insulin-dependent diabetes mellitus (NIDDM). Type 1 diabetes, also known as juvenile-onset diabetes, is typified by an absolute insulin deficiency thought to be caused by an auto-immune response to nonspecific viral infections of the beta cells of the pancreas. The disease is usually detected before the age of 30 (C. Thomas 1997, 529). Type 2 diabetes, also known as adult-onset diabetes, is closely associated with obesity and involves a gradual decline in the quantity of insulin produced by the pancreas with associated resistance to insulin in the peripheral tissues (Weiss et al. 1989). Until recently, it was rarely found in individuals under the age of forty and can usually be controlled by dietary changes. While Type 1 diabetes is rarely found in Native Americans, rates of Type 2 diabetes are exceptionally high with age-adjusted diabetes mortality rates among Native Americans nationwide at 2.5 times the rate of the general U.S. population in 1980 (Young 1996; Gohdes, Kaufman, and Valway 1993). The Pima Indians, who exhibit the highest rates of Type 2 diabetes in the world, have a prevalence of around 50 percent for adults over age thirty-five (Boyce and Swinburn 1993).

Diabetes is associated with increased risk for a wide range of conditions and, while it was the sixth underlying cause of death among Native Americans between 1984 and 1986, it is a contributing factor for other causes of death and disease (Gohdes, Kaufman, and Valway 1993). Impaired vascular circulation slows the healing of wounds in peripheral areas, and minor foot injuries, unnoticed due to loss of feeling in extremities, can quickly lead to infection and often amputation (Weiss et al. 1989). Visual problems leading to blindness are associated with advanced diabetes. Diabetic retinopathy, a result of hemorrhaging in the retina, is quickly becoming the leading cause of adult blindness in the United States, with rates estimated to be as much as twenty-five times higher than that of nondiabetics (Ferris 1993). Cataracts are also more than twice as likely to occur among diabetics as nondiabetics (Reinhard and Greenwalt 1975). Diabetes also has a deleterious effect on the kidneys, advancing to total kidney failure or End-Stage Renal Disease (ESRD). Nearly 60 percent of all ESRD cases among Native Americans are associated with diabetes. The incidence of ESRD among Native Americans is three times that of whites, while among Native Americans with diabetes the incidence increases to six times that of whites (Young 1996).

Other complications associated with diabetes include cardiovascular disease, periodontal disease, increased susceptibility to tuberculosis, decreased cognitive function (Lowe et al. 1994), and an increased prevalence of arthritis, gallstones, benign and malignant tumors, and hypertension (Reinhard and Greenwalt 1975). Cardiovascular disease rates, which were generally lower in Native Americans than in the general population, have been increasing due to increased urbanization and adoption of the standard American diet (Gillum et al. 1984). Even among groups in which rates tend to be lower, such as the Navajo (Welty and Coulehan 1993), 50 percent of all heart patients were also diagnosed with Type 2 diabetes (Gohdes, Kaufman, and Valway 1993). Rates of periodontal disease among Pima Indians over thirty-five years old are more than five times greater in diabetics than in nondiabetics (Loe 1993). High rates and increasing incidence of tuberculosis can also be directly attributed to diabetes, with latent infections becoming active due to compromised immune function associated with diabetes (Wilkins 1996; Rieder 1989; Snipp 1996; Breault 1997).

Early investigations of the prevalence of diabetes among the Eastern Cherokee showed that rates of the disease were exceptionally high (Stein et al. 1965). More recently, it was confirmed that as many as 25 percent of the adults over thirty-five years old are diabetics, and there is a direct correlation of disease rate to percentage of Indian heritage. While only 28 percent of the total population registered as having a minimum of 75 percent Indian heritage, 60 percent of the diabetic patients were found to be above that threshold. This translates to a nearly fourfold increase in the rate of diabetes for those having a minimum of 75 percent Indian heritage. This is comparable to the three- to fivefold increase found among full-inheritance individuals of the Choctaw and the Three Affiliated Tribes when compared to those of mixed heritage (Weiss, Ferrell, and Hanis 1984). Rates of complication in Cherokee patients that were attributed to diabetes were also exceptionally high. Lower-extremity amputation rates were three times higher in Cherokee diabetic patients when compared to all racial groups in the United States in 1978. This rate is comparable to rates among the Pima Indians, known to have the highest rates of diabetes of any group in North America. Hypertension effects Cherokee diabetics at a rate of 53 percent, slightly higher than the 47.5 percent rate for Navajo diabetics but comparable to the general population in the United States (Farrell et al. 1993). ESRD rates among the Cherokee from 1983 to 1986 were 2.5 times higher than rates for all American Indian populations (Quiggins and Farrell 1993).

The earliest explanatory model for a genetic origin for the prevalence of diabetes among Native Americans, first proposed in 1962, was Neel's "thrifty genotype" hypothesis. According to Neel, the first immigrants to the North American continent were hunter-gatherers who lived for thousands of years in the harsh environments of Siberia and Alaska and would have experienced alternating periods of food scarcity and abundance. Those who carried a genetic makeup that allowed them to store excess calories as fat for times of shortage had a selective advantage during periods of famine. They would also have had the added benefit of a protective fat layer for survival in the Arctic conditions endured during the migration to North America (Weiss et al. 1989).

Hyperinsulinemia, which facilitates fat storage, would have been a selective advantage during periods of feast or famine. Apparently supporting a genetic explanation, it was observed that Native American groups in the Southwest have demonstrated higher insulin levels than their white counterparts under similar dietary regimens (Sievers and Fisher 1981). The tendency to efficiently store excess calories would cease to be a selective advantage under contemporary conditions of a constant food supply. The logical conclusion is that the genetic predisposition, combined with a move away from traditional diets and active lifestyles, has led to the present rates of obesity and diabetes.

Szathmary has proposed an alternative hypothesis based on her studies of the Dogrib tribe in Canada's Northwest Territories. Assuming that the conditions present when Asiatic peoples entered North America were similar to those present today in northern Canada, Szathmary suggests that selective pressures favored individuals who could efficiently subsist on a diet low in carbohydrates, high in protein, and with a moderate amount of fat (Szathmary 1986). The efficient processing and storage of glucose synthesized from other biological sources such as protein would be an advantage in a region of limited, seasonal availability of plant foods. The conclusion from this hypothesis is the same as that of the "thrifty genotype" hypothesis: an adaptation that once provided selective advantage is detrimental under current lifestyle conditions.

Changes in diet that would have occurred with migration to the south and increased consumption of plant foods would still have kept the incidence of metabolic diseases low. The incorporation of agricultural practices that led to the domestication of corn, beans, and squash would have increased the carbohydrate content of the diet. While nutritional status was decreased as a result of this diet, the high energy content of these foods was essential to meet the increased workloads associated with agriculture. Both the increased muscular activity associated with agricultural practices and the high fiber content of the vegetable products that would slow absorption from the intestines would decrease the need for insulin. The ability to easily store fat would still be advantageous during times of famine and seasonal shortages (Ritenbaugh and Goodby 1989).

Because of the strength of the statistical evidence for a genetic etiology for the metabolic disorders associated with diabetes, the thrifty gene hypothesis and its offspring are nearly universally accepted as an explanation for higher rates of obesity and diabetes in Native Americans. However, the impressive numbers may have biased researchers to accept the hypothesis as fact. Some are beginning to question the underlying energetic and selective assumptions of the hypothesis. For instance, the assumption that hunter-gatherers are more prone to famine events than agriculturalists has been challenged by ethnographic and historical comparisons between both groups, which suggests that the opposite may be more accurate. Sedentary agriculturalists tend to be more reliant on a narrower range of foods than hunter-gatherers, making them more vulnerable during a famine event (Cordain, Miller, and Mann 1999; Benyshek and Watson 2006).

There are also concerns as to whether the frequency of famine events or their effect on a population would trigger the selection suggested in the thrifty gene hypothesis. Famines generally occur at intervals of 100 to 150 years, too long an interval for efficient fat deposition to display any selective advantage, and mortality rates rarely exceed 10 percent of the population. Mortality is usually due to disease, not starvation, with little differentiation in rates between lean and obese individuals (Speakman 2006). It has also been pointed out that in spite of over forty years of genetic research attempting to identify the "thrifty gene," no promising candidate has been identified (Speakman 2006; McDermott 1998).

Changing demographics across all racial and age groups also indicate that increasing rates of metabolic disorders are a global phenomenon independent of racial boundaries. The prevalence of diabetes has generally been higher in the indigenous populations living in developed countries (Yeats and Tonelli 2006); however, the shift toward parity is alarming. The rate of obese and overweight adults in the United States is now greater than 60 percent, and rates for children and adolescents tripled between 1980 and 2000 (Wyatt, Winters, and Dubbert 2006). Other industrialized nations, such as Taiwan, the United Kingdom, Australia, and New Zealand, are experiencing similar trends toward obesity with associated increases in rates for diabetes (Tseng et al. 2006; McMahon et al. 2004; Hotu et al. 2004). Developing nations such as India and China are also experiencing sharp increases in diabetes rates, and projections for 2025 suggest that up to 75 percent of the estimated 300,000 diabetes cases will be in the developing nations (Mohan 2004). The short time span for the alarming increase in rates of obesity and related metabolic disorders, a matter of a few decades, is much too short of a period to indicate a genetic change in all populations and indicates that the cause for such changes is environmental (Ailhaud et al. 2006). The statistical anomalies for Native Americans appear to be more anecdotal evidence than definitive explanations for supporting a genetic etiology for diabetes, and perhaps such numbers explain more of a "canary-in-the-coal-mine" phenomenon than a genetic predisposition.

In closing this section, I would like to consider just one of a number of hypothetical environmental explanations for the exceptional statistics that formed and inspired the basis of the thrifty gene hypothesis. Weiss et al. (1984) indicate that African Americans and Native Americans share a similar socioeconomic status, but Native Americans have higher rates of metabolic disorders. However, comparable socioeconomic status does not automatically translate into an ability to make comparable life choices. African Americans are several generations removed from the type of social control exhibited and continuing on Indian reservations.

For instance, Native American reservations were strictly controlled by the U.S. government and the inhabitants were early recipients of supplementary foods that later became government commodities programs. The initial offerings generally often consisted of nothing more than flour, salt, sugar, coffee, and oil or lard. Commodities are notorious for being high in fat, salt, and processed carbohydrates (Dillinger et al. 1999). Recognition of the relationship between commodity consumption and obesity was observed in Native American communities and was labeled with the term "Comod Bod" (Welty 1991). The residual evidence of the prevalence of commodities is the ubiquitous frybread, a staple food in Native American homes and festivals across the United States and Canada (Smith and Wiedman 2001). While frybread has become a symbol of unity and pride among Native Americans, it is also a relic of government patrimony, which led to the loss of traditional dietary practices and higher rates of obesity (Harjo 2005).

Frybread is not solely responsible for the high rates of metabolic disorders among Native Americans, but it is indicative of the types of environmental factors that must be explored regardless of whether the "thrifty gene" is ever identified. Diabetes was not a common affliction of the Native American community until after World War II (Dillinger et al. 1999), indicating that something had changed a generation or so before the war to trigger an epidemic of metabolic disorders. No preventive approach to the pandemic of diabetes will be successful without examining the changes that were common across cultures in the latter half of the twentieth century.

Perhaps the recent surge in the condemnation of trans fatty acids for their implicated role in cardiovascular disease, systemic inflammation, cancer, and diabetes will provide part of an explanation (Mozaffarian et al. 2006; Odegaard and Pereira 2006; Riserus 2006). Trans fats were introduced to the public on a grand scale during World War II as a solution to a butter shortage in the form of margarine and shortening. If the postwar surpluses of products laden with partially hydrogenated vegetable oils were distributed as part of the supplemental food program to the reservations, negative effects would have been obvious in a relatively short time. The inclusion of lard and shortening in the USDA Food Assistance Programs starting in the late 1960s (Feeley and Watt 1970) and the increasing frequency of the use of partially hydrogenated vegetable oil in most commercially prepared foods and the fast foods by the mid-1980s would have spread diabetes and associated metabolic disorders throughout the nation and the world, well beyond the borders of the reservations.

Trans fatty acids may not be the primary factor that led to the proliferation of diabetes, but until environmental factors like the dietary increase in trans fats after World War II are fully considered it is unproductive and possibly detrimental to pursue a purely genetic explanation. As a recent study of the Pima has demonstrated, genetically similar populations on either side of the border between Mexico and the United States have radically different rates of obesity and diabetes (Schultz et al. 2006). The fivefold increase in rates for Pima living on the U.S. side of the border strongly implicates the living environment. Accepting the fate of a genetic predisposition toward a chronic illness such as diabetes diminishes the incentive to critically examine social, historical, and environmental conditions and dilutes the effectiveness of disease prevention programs that promote lifestyle changes or deeper psychosocial examination (Liburd et al. 2006; McDermott 1999).

## Cholelithiasis

Cholelithiasis, or the formation and presence of gallstones, is a result of excess caloric intake. There is a direct correlation between levels of obesity and the incidence of gallstones (Mendez-Sanchez et al. 2005). Gallstones appear when the bile becomes supersaturated with cholesterol, which precipitates out and coagulates to form stones. High insulin levels of the sort found in both obese individuals and those with gallstones stimulate cholesterol synthesis (Maclure et al. 1988). Obesity also produces a state of hypocontractility in the gallbladder (Tran et al. 2003), which promotes a condition of stasis of bile and creates a favorable environment for stone formation (Nakeeb et al. 2006; Andersen 1992). The consumption of legumes has also been implicated in the formation of gallstones (Nervi et al. 1989); however, this appears not to pertain to Native Americans, as they have been consuming legumes for many generations previous to any record of complications (Sievers and Fisher 1981) and Asians, who consume a legume-rich diet, have a low propensity for gallstones (Weiss et al. 1984).

The close association of gallstone formation with diabetes suggests a common etiology. Hyperinsulinemia associated with obesity is common to both, as is sensitivity to carbohydrates, especially readily available carbohydrates. The change from lightly processed, traditional foods to highly processed, refined carbohydrate sources eliminates the modifying effect of dietary fiber and increases the rate of uptake of sugars (Heaton 1984). Diabetics are almost twice as likely as nondiabetics to be afflicted with gallstones (Mendez-Sanchez 2005; Caroli et al. 2004).

Native Americans have exceptionally high rates of biliary disease and, as a result of the pervasiveness of gallstones, they have been called the "American Indian's burden" (Sievers and Fisher 1981). However, as with diabetes, the prevalence of gallstones seems to be a contemporary problem associated with a Westernized lifestyle and dietary changes. Early reports on Indian health matters made no mention of biliary diseases (Shaheb 1990). In Daniel Moerman's *Native American Ethnobotany* (2003), which contains over 44,000 entries of uses for 2,147 species of plants used by 123 groups, there are only eight references to plants used for gallstones. The conspicuous absence of gallstone remedies in traditional Native American medicine is testimony for the recent development of the condition.

As with diabetes, the high statistical representation of gallstones among Native Americans provided anecdotal evidence for a genetic basis for gallbladder disease. The premise is similar to the thrifty gene hypothesis: embracing a Westernized lifestyle exacerbates the genetic predisposition for certain conditions. But, just as in the case of diabetes, the evidence remains anecdotal as no human susceptibility genes have been identified for gallbladder disease (Everhart et al. 2002).

Rates of gallbladder disease, just like those of diabetes, are rising among all racial groups and approaching parity with Native American rates. Two decades ago it was determined that women were more susceptible to gallstones than were men, having rates two to three times that of men among Caucasians and four to five times the frequency in Native Americans (Weiss et al. 1984). More recent literature surveys now conclude that the ratio of women to men with gallbladder disease across racial lines is approaching 4:1 (Nakeeb et al. 2002). Racial parity is evident in other groups, including identical rates for Hispanic and Mapuche Indian men in Chile and for Mexican American and non-Hispanic white men in the United States (Everhart et al. 2002).

There has been some correlation between the long-term intake of trans fatty acids and gallstone formation, with trans fat consumers showing a modest increase in the rate of gallbladder disease (Tsai et al. 2005). However, the cohort in this study consisted of well-educated health professionals who would have access to superior dietary choices when compared to populations from lower socioeconomic categories (Drewnowski and Specter 2004). Higher socioeconomic status is associated with a higher consumption of fruits and vegetables, a factor that appears to lower the risk of gallbladder disease (Tsai et al. 2006).

## Cervical Cancer

Until very recently, Native Americans had demonstrated consistently lower rates of cancer than those of the general population. A comparison of rates for all cancer mortalities for Native Americans from 1989 through 1991 and the general U.S. population in 1990 showed that the rate for Native Americans was 30 percent less than that of the general population (Young 1996).

However, recent statistics suggest that rates are climbing, and cancer is now the second leading cause of death among Native Americans (Farmer, Bell, and Stark 2005).

While Native American rates of cancer of the breast, lung, and colon have been significantly lower than those of the total U.S. population, others such as cancer of the kidney in men and gallbladder and cervix in women are substantially higher (Young 1996). For instance, mortality rates between 1984 and 1988 for cervical cancer for Native American women were at 7.6 per 100,000, compared to 3.1 per 100,000 for all U.S. women. Among Native American women in the southeastern United States, mortality rates for the same period were 11.6 per 100,000 (Dignan et al. 1994). Health education programs designed to detect and treat cervical cancer improved these figures, with mortality rates in the 1989 to 1993 period at 3.0 per 100,000 in the general population and 5.8 per 100,000 in Native American women. The most dramatic decrease was among southeastern Native American women, where mortality rates dropped to 3.1 per 100,000 (Messer, Steckler, and Dignan 1999). In the Cherokee community, the success of the program was attributed to three factors. First, the establishment of the Women's Evening Clinic provided an easy-access, woman-friendly environment for cervical cancer screening. The clinic was staffed by women practitioners and opened in the evenings with day care facilities. Second, large numbers of women attended the Cherokee Hospital Diabetes Clinic and were encouraged by doctors to get annual cervical cancer screenings. Third, the Cherokee community is very close-knit and interrelated, and deaths attributed to cancer raise community awareness of the problem (Messer, Steckler, and Dignan 1999). These factors help overcome women's reserve in dealing with such a personal topic and their reluctance to seek medical attention with no evident symptoms.

The etiology of cervical cancer is related to a number of factors, including the age of first sexual intercourse and number of sexual partners, cigarette smoking, use of oral contraceptives, and dietary factors. The number of sexual partners is implicated in elevated risk for cervical cancer through an increased risk for infection with the human papillomavirus (HPV), possibility of infection with multiple HPV strains (Ho et al. 1998), and contact with male penile cancer (Reeves et al. 1989). Cigarette smoking depletes bodily reserves of Vitamin C and carotenoids. The anti-oxidants Vitamins A, C, and E are associated with a reduced risk of all stages of cervical cancer and also helped lower risk among HPV positive individuals (Potischman 1993; Ho et al. 1998; Herrero et al. 1991). Carotenoids, such as beta-carotene and lycopene, have been shown to be preventive against a range of cancers, with lycopene demonstrating the most beneficial deterrent effect for cervical cancer (Bendich 1989; Brock et al. 1988; J. Olson 1989; Mascio, Kaiser, and Sies 1989; Clinton 1998). Oral contraceptive use, especially in the long term, may deplete the body's reserves of folate, a potential deterrent against the early stages of cervical cancer (Butterworth et al. 1992; Kim 1999).

While more research into nutritional factors affecting cervical and other forms of cancer is needed, there is strong evidence that a diet high in fruits and vegetables had an inverse relationship to the rate of all cancers (Ziegler 1989). This may be due to higher levels of intake of carotenoids, Vitamin C, or folate, a combination of these factors, or intrinsic factors not yet identified. The mechanism is still unknown, yet it is clear that increasing dietary intake of fruits and vegetables is an important factor in lowering the risk for cervical cancer (Giuliano 2000; Key 1994).

## Applying Traditional Cherokee Foods

Understanding the present Cherokee situation requires reflecting on the history of the last two hundred years. Acculturation of portions of the Cherokee tribe was well under way by 1800, especially in the southern end of the Cherokee lands in the northern parts of Georgia and Alabama and in eastern Tennessee. Many prominent citizens, a high percentage of whom were mixed white/Cherokee heritage, owned and operated large plantations, and the most affluent owned slaves to work their lands. These plantations were indistinguishable from those belonging to their white counterparts as were the products raised on them. However, in the mountainous region of western North Carolina, the conservative element of Cherokee society was dominant. They tended to be full-blood Cherokee and were more resistant to accepting European customs and language. The farms in this region were traditionally much smaller and had significantly lower yields than those of other parts of the Cherokee lands because of topography and poor soils (McLoughlin and Conser 1977).

Culinary aspects of acculturation were mixed among the Cherokee. The deerskin trade of the eighteenth century reduced the availability of venison, which resulted in a depletion of other game animals and dependence on European livestock. The Cherokee were slow to embrace cattle, especially in regions with limited pasturage. But with the collapse of the deerskin trade around 1790, the raising of cattle and horses became an important means for Cherokee men to ensure the flow of needed European trade items (Waselkov 1997). However, pigs and chickens could be fed on garden wastes and became an adjunct to gardening for Cherokee women. By 1900, domesticated animals were well incorporated into the Cherokee diet and the paucity of low-fat game animals resulted in an increased consumption of high-fat pork (Finger 1991, 8).

Several plant foods were readily incorporated into Cherokee gardens and orchards. The Spanish introduced sweet potatoes (*Ipomoea batatas*), peaches (*Prunus persica*), and watermelons (*Citrullus lanatus*) to the southeastern Indians, and these were well established in Cherokee villages when the English began exploring the area (Hatley 1991).

The region of North Carolina where the Eastern Band of the Cherokee remained is in one of the most biologically diverse temperate zone forests in the world. A relatively short growing season due to the higher altitudes is a limiting factor for agricultural production, but this is easily offset by an abundance of wild or semi-cultivated foods. The Cherokee had a wide selection of floral and faunal food sources to augment traditional foods and introduced crops and livestock. The remainder of this chapter will focus on the relationship of the traditional Cherokee dietary regime to diabetes, gallbladder disease, and cervical cancer.

## Animal Foods

Animal foods in the traditional Cherokee diet provided a good source of protein with little fat. The major game animals (bears, deer, rabbits, and squirrels) were supplemented by several consistently reliable minor animal foods. Small birds were hunted with blowguns or caught in traps, roasted, cleaned, and added to soups. Small fish were dried by the fire and cooked with corn as a breakfast mush. Box turtles were roasted in their shells and eaten from the shell or in soups (Witthoft n.d., 159–60). The traditional cooking techniques of boiling or roasting animal foods would have kept the fat content low. Some have even speculated that the game animals of the Eastern Woodlands were so deficient in fat content that nuts were an essential source of calories in the late winter months (Gardner 1997).

The introduction of pigs would have increased the availability of lard, and cast iron skillets made frying an option for preparing foods. However, these changes in cooking techniques have been with the Cherokee for over 250 years and obesity seems to be a more recent phenomenon. While additional fat may exacerbate the problem of obesity and the associated conditions of diabetes and gallstones, it is only a part of the current problem and must be considered in light of changing levels of physical activity. Dietary fat has been linked to an increase in levels of sex hormones and associated with an increase in risk for estrogen-dependent cancers (Boik 1996, 131), but it is still unclear whether it is a factor in cervical cancer.

One change that occurred in the quality of fat consumed in the twentieth century was the transformation from free-ranging hogs to feedlot animals. Cherokee hogs were semi-wild and allowed to forage in the mountains until they were well fattened by the fall acorn and chestnut mast. The final product was a leaner hog that may have had a more favorable fatty acid profile. Recent studies show that hogs, fish, and chickens fed on a diet rich in omega-3 fatty acids had a higher content of omega-3 fatty acids in their flesh and in the eggs of the chickens, as well as a more favorable ration of omega-3 to omega-6 fatty acids (Karapanagiotidis et al. 2006; Millet et al. 2006; Ailhaud et al. 2006). Nuts in general are a good source of omega-3 fatty acids (Simopoulos 2006), and the lard of semi-wild Cherokee hogs would have had a much higher ratio of omega-3 to omega-6 fatty acids than feedlot hogs raised on a predominantly corn-based diet. Diets high in omega-6 fatty acids have been indicated in the deposition of excessive adipose tissue (Ailhaud et al. 2006), adding to the range of factors causing obesity. It may be that the establishment of the Great Smoky Mountains National Park in the 1930s, when the Cherokee were forced to confine their hogs in pens, limited the availability of nut mast and changed the quality of the lard used in Cherokee cooking. The subsequent change from an agriculturally based economy to a predominantly tourist-oriented economy would have increased the dependence on commercially produced pork products and caused further erosion in the quality of the Cherokee diet.

## Agricultural Products

The primary traditional crops of Native North America, corn (*Zea mays*), beans (*Phaseolus vulgaris*), and squash (*Cucurbita spp.*), would have been excellent foods for preventing the diseases considered here and all were important in the Cherokee diet. A favorite Cherokee method of preparing corn is to make bean-bread. Corn meal is added to cooked beans, chestnuts or other nuts, or fresh berries and pounded into stiff dough. The mixture is then wrapped in a corn leaf and cooked like dumplings in boiling water (Witthoft n.d., 187). Corn prepared in this fashion provides a good source of complex carbohydrates and dietary fiber, which helps regulate the absorption of glucose. Corn has also been shown to exhibit a hypoglycemic activity, but the active constituent has yet to be identified (Bever and Zhand 1979).

The majority of Native American groups that depended on corn as a major component of subsistence included some form of alkali processing at some stage of preparation (Katz et al. 1975). This was true for the traditional Cherokee method of corn preparation, which included the use of ashes from the cooking fire, preferably from hickory wood, in the initial process of soaking and hulling the corn (Witthoft n.d., 154, 189). Alkali processing imparts several nutritional benefits to corn, including an increase in the availability of niacin, tryptophan, and lysine, as well as the inactivation of fungal toxins that are produced on stored grain (Katz, Hediger, and Valleroy 1975; Bressini 1990).

Beans have played an important role in traditional dietary practices around the world, but they suffer from an image problem and have been referred to as the "poor man's meat." They are an excellent source of folate and provide a good source of complex carbohydrates and fiber, especially soluble fiber, which has been shown to reduce blood sugar and cholesterol levels (Messina 1999). Beans are also considered to be antidiabetic because of the organic sulphides contained in them. These are thought to bind to insulin-inactivating compounds and thus have a sparing effect on insulin (Bever and Zhand 1979). Beans also exhibit a weak estrogenic effect that may be beneficial in preventing estrogen-dependent cancers (Messina 1999).

Pumpkins and squash, especially the yellow-fleshed winter variety, are an excellent source of beta-carotene and would be a preventive factor against cervical cancer. One of the Cherokee favorites was the candy roaster squash, a large squash with green, white, and orange colorings on the skin. Large squashes were prepared by either roasting or boiling, but pumpkins were often sliced into a large spiral resembling an apple peel and dried by the fire for storage (Witthoft n.d., 200–201).

Many of the introduced crop species are now known to demonstrate a preventive role against various forms of cancer. Sweet potatoes are comparable to winter squash in their beta-carotene content (Robertson, Flinders, and Ruppenthal 1986, 468). Watermelon is a good source of Vitamin C and, as mentioned earlier, is high in the carotenoid lycopene. Lycopene exhibits a strong anti-oxidant capacity and appears to be effective in preventing the proliferation of several forms of cancer cells, including those of cervical cancer (Clinton 1998; "Lycopene" 2003). Cabbage (*Brassica oleracea*, var. *capitata*), introduced to the Cherokee by the British, is known to exhibit a wide range of biological activities that can potentially inhibit the onset of cancer (Beecher 1994).

## Wild Foods

The medicinal properties of the wild and semi-cultivated foods used by the Cherokee are even more impressive than those reported for agricultural products. Wild foods are used worldwide to supplement both macronutrient (protein, carbohydrates, and lipids) and micronutrient (vitamins and minerals) needs. The high micronutrient content of wild foods can balance a diet limited in macronutrients and ensure good health in the face of macronutrient deficiency (Grivetti and Ogle 2000). The collection of wild foods is a coping strategy during times of famine (Corbett 1988), and wild vegetables are often the primary vegetable products consumed in many parts of the world, even when their domestic counterparts are available (Grivetti and Ogle 2000).

The spring brought a variety of fresh greens to the Cherokee table. Green leafy plants in general tend to be a good source of folate (Segura et al. 2006), discussed above as a possible preventive agent for the formation of cervical dysplasia (Butterworth et al. 1992). Certain greens like the creasy greens (*Barbarea vulgaris* and *B. verna*) and sochana (*Rudbeckia lacinata*) were some of the first available in the spring. Though little is known about the nutritional value of sochana, creasy greens share the same anti-cancer properties as other members of the cabbage family (*Brassicaceae*) and contain more than two and one half times the Vitamin C of oranges (Zennie and Ogzewalla 1977). Several other introduced and native members of this family were incorporated into the Cherokee diet, such as pepper grass (*Lepidium virginicum*), bitter cress (*Cardamine pensylvanica*), several species of toothwort (*Dentaria spp.*), and shepherd's purse (*Capsella bursa-pastoris*) (Witthoft 1977). All members of the family *Brassicaceae* are known to contain the organic sulphides mentioned above as hypoglycemic and anti-cancer agents (Bever and Zhand 1979).

A little later in the spring the young shoots of pokeweed (*Phytolacca americana*) are harvested and relished by the Cherokee. The early growth is best harvested when the plants are six to eight inches tall and are boiled in two changes of water to remove the toxic saponins (Duke 1992, 148). Pokeweed was used as a folk remedy for cancer (Crellin and Philpott 1989, 350) and contains a protein known as pokeweed antiviral protein (PAP), which demonstrated a significant inhibitory effect against viral infection by the influenza virus, poliovirus, and the herpes simplex virus (Teltow, Irvin, and Aron 1983). Whether this antiviral property would apply to HPV remains to be determined.

Ramps (*Allium tricoccum*) are also gathered in the early spring and the portion above the bulb is prepared by parboiling in changes of water (Witthoft n.d., 26). Those who indulge in eating raw ramps can be identified for several days by their odor (Chiltoskey 1975), which is due to the organic sulphides. While no studies have been performed directly on the beneficial

qualities of ramps, they have been shown to contain many of the same or-
ganosulfur compounds as the closely related onion (*Allium cepa*) and garlic
(*Allium sativum*). Both onions and garlic have been shown to significantly
lower blood sugar levels (Mukherjee et al. 2006) and prevent a wide range of
cancers (Wargovich 1999). Ramps are also an excellent source of Vitamin C,
having around 80 milligrams per 100 grams (Zennie and Ogzewalla 1977), or
nearly double the amount found in oranges.

Many of the wild greens eaten by the Cherokee are the weedy species
associated with their gardens and farm fields during the summer months.
Lambs-quarters (*Chenopodium album*) may be one of the most nutritious,
having between 12,000 and 14,000 IU of Vitamin A and 130 milligrams of
Vitamin C per 100 grams (Zennie and Ogzewalla 1977). Later in the season the black nightshade (*Solanum nigrum*) becomes available. Touted as a
favorite green of the Cherokee (Cozzo 2004, 254), the edible greens are relished in many parts of the world (Defelice 2003). Of seventy wild plant
foods tested in India, *Solanum nigrum* proved to have the highest total carotenoid content and had the highest levels of beta-carotene (Rajyalakshmi
et al. 2001).

Starting in early summer several types of wild berries are available in the
southern Appalachian Mountains. Strawberries (*Fragaria virginiana*) and
service berries (*Amelanchier arborea*) were the first to appear, followed by
mulberries (*Morus rubra*) and black raspberries (*Rubus occidentalis*), then the
blackberries and raspberries (*Rubus spp.*). By late summer and into the fall,
the elderberries (*Sambucus canadensis*), blueberries (*Vaccinium spp.*), huckle-
berries (*Gaylussacia spp.*), and several species of wild grapes (*Vitis spp.*) were
available. Berries were generally eaten fresh in the field or were cooked in
cornbread to give it added flavor. The traditional storage method, before
the introduction of canning and freezing, was to dry berries for future use.
Grapes were dried in clusters around the cooking hearth and boiled during
the winter to make a beverage (Witthoft n.d., 40–45).

Berries in general are good sources of a wide range of anti-oxidants, many
complementing each other and enhancing the cumulative anti-oxidant effect (Scalzo, Mezzetti, and Battino 2005). Some of the most beneficial anti-
oxidants in berries include the anthocyanins and ellagitannins. Anthocyanins are flavanoid pigments that give the coloring to black, blue, and red
fruits, and are especially concentrated in the darker fruits. As a group, anthocyanins tend to have an anti-oxidative capacity much higher than Vitamin C (Ariga 2004). Blueberries, several species of which are common to
the southern Appalachian region, are especially high in anti-oxidant nutri-

ents (Kalt et al. 1999; Prior et al. 1998); however, the low-bush varieties have a higher total anti-oxidant capacity than the high-bush varieties (Kalt et al. 2001). The bramble fruits (blackberries, black raspberries, and red raspberries), elderberries, and service berries are all noted for their high anthocyanin content and excellent anti-oxidant capacity (Sellappan, Akoh, and Krewer 2002; Liu et al. 2005; Wada and Ou 2002; Beekwilder, Hall, and de Vos 2005; "*Sambucus nigra*" 2005; Adhikari et al. 2005).

Anthocyanins as a group display a wide range of biological activities, many of which are beneficial for diabetics and for cancer prevention. In animal studies, anthocyanins stimulated pancreatic cells to secrete insulin (Jayaprakasam et al. 2005) and demonstrated an inhibitory effect on the factors in fat cells that can lead to obesity and insulin resistance (Tsuda et al. 2005). Anthocyanins have also been shown to maintain vascular permeability (Youdim et al. 2000), which would aid with the circulatory problems associated with diabetes. This would be especially helpful with microvascular problems of the eyes, such as the complications associated with diabetic retinopathy. Anthocyanins have also demonstrated the potential to resist macular degeneration (Jang et al. 2005).

The anti-oxidant properties of anthocyanins would lend support to other factors in fruits and vegetables that aid in preventing cervical cancer. Anthocyanins suppressed the growth and proliferation of a wide variety of cancer cells, including those associated with cancer of the uterus, breast, lungs, and colon, and consumption of large amounts of strawberries cut the rate of all types of cancer in elderly individuals to nearly one-third of the rate experienced by those who did not regularly eat them (Cooke et al. 2005).

The other class of anti-oxidants in berries that exhibit a powerful beneficial effect are the ellagitannins, dietary polyphenols consisting of ellagic acid subunits. Ellagitannins are especially prevalent in raspberries and strawberries (Cerdá, Tomás-Barberán, and Espín 2005; Mullen et al. 2002). Various ellagitannins have been found to inhibit mutations that initiate cancer-causing cell damage, prevent the formation of cancerous tumors, and enhance the immune response against existing tumors (Okuda, Yoshida, and Hatano 1988).

Fall was the season to harvest nuts and wild roots. Hickory nuts (*Carya spp.*), black walnuts (*Juglans nigra*), acorns (*Quercus alba*), and chestnuts (*Castanea americana*) were traditional fall fare for the Cherokee and all were added to cornbread. Acorn use fell off around 1890 and the chestnut blight destroyed the entire crop by the mid-1950s. However, hickory nuts and black walnuts are still available. Hickory nuts were generally crushed in the shell in corn mortars and the resulting paste rolled into a ball. This was dropped in boiling water where the shells would settle to the bottom and the resulting milk was used as a base for soups, drunk as a beverage, or added to cornbread. Walnuts were removed from the shells and eaten raw or crushed and boiled to separate the oil. This oil, which was later superseded by hog lard, was at one time the only cooking oil available to the Cherokee (Witthoft n.d., 46–48, 51–52).

The inclusion of nuts in the diet provides a high-energy food that exhibits a range of beneficial effects on the consumer. Regular consumption of nuts was found to lower the risk of coronary heart disease and decreased levels of total cholesterol as well as low-density lipoprotein cholesterol (Drehler, Maher, and Kearney 1996). While the nuts specific to the traditional Cherokee diet have not been extensively studied for their beneficial effects, nuts in general are being touted as very desirable food for diabetics. Consumption of nuts helps regulate blood glucose levels and decrease insulin sensitivity in people with Type 2 diabetes (Rajaram and Sabate 2006). Another nutritional benefit of nuts is their high magnesium content, which appears to be closely associated with the risk of developing diabetes (Lopez-Ridaura et al. 2004; McCarty 2005). Nuts are also a good source of omega-3 fatty acids. A decrease in the ratio of omega-6 to omega-3 fatty acids in the diet decreases the inflammatory response that leads to chronic diseases such as diabetes and heart disease (Simopoulos 2006) and may have a beneficial effect on the depression that often accompanies Type 2 diabetes (Pouwer et al. 2005). English walnuts, a close relative of the black walnuts and hickory nuts used by the Cherokee, are specifically being recommended for diabetics because of their high omega-3 fatty acid content and favorable polyunsaturated fatty acid profile (Gillen et al. 2005). Thirty grams of walnuts per day had a beneficial effect on cholesterol levels and the ratio of HDL cholesterol to total cholesterol level in diabetic patients, reducing their risk of coronary disease (Tapsell et al. 2004).

Nuts are also a good source of folate, a possible factor in the prevention of cervical cancer (Drehler, Maher, and Kearney 1996). As mentioned above, low blood levels of folate may be associated with an increase in the risk factors associated with cervical dysplasia, especially infection with the human papillomavirus (Butterworth et al. 1992). Nuts, especially walnuts (Cerdá, Tomás-Barberán, and Espín 2005), are a good source of ellagitannins, already discussed above for their role in cancer prevention. The traditional method of eating greens with nut oil poured on them would have been nutritionally superior to the later practice of replacing nut oil with hog grease.

Frequent nut consumption was also found to significantly lower the risk of gallbladder disease in both men and women (Tsai et al. 2004a, 2004b). The high content of unsaturated fatty acids, which would replace saturated and trans fatty acids, leads to lowered cholesterol levels, thus reducing gall-stone formation. The same studies found an inverse relationship between the consumption of nuts and increases in body mass. Nut consumers tend to weigh less than non-consumers, possibly a result of the ability of nuts to satisfy the consumer's appetite and craving for less desirable foods.

Fall was also the season to dig root crops for winter storage. Two of the several wild root crops reported to be used by the Cherokee are relevant to this discussion. Groundnut (*Apios americana*) produces several egg-sized tubers along each root. These are boiled and eaten or mashed and incorporated into cornbread (Witthoft n.d., 34). The aerial portion also produces small beans that were used in making bean-bread (Perry 1974, 46). The root and bean contain the isoflavone daidzein, which weakens the estrogenic effect. Daidzein binds to estrogen receptor sites and inhibits the stronger effects of estrogen, which exacerbates many forms of cancer (Newmark 1996, 31).

Jerusalem artichoke (*Helianthus tuberosus*) produces copious amounts of small tubers that were eaten raw, boiled, or baked by the Cherokee (Witthoft n.d., 34). Jerusalem artichokes are high in inulin, a polysaccharide that consists of long chains of fructose instead of the glucose found in starches (Pengelly 1997, 42). Inulin reduces the risk of Type 2 diabetes and obesity, apparently through its effects on lipid metabolism and adjustments of insulin levels (Roberfroid and Delzenne 1998), as well as through its ability to lower blood glucose levels (Rumessen et al. 1990). Inulin is considered to have a prebiotic effect, causing the intestinal flora balance to shift toward beneficial bacteria that increase fecal bulk and improve intestinal motility (Roberfroid 1999), which would aid in problems with gallbladder stasis. More research is necessary to determine the extent of the health benefits of inulin and other fructose-based polysaccharides.

## Conclusion

The Cherokee are faced with environmental limitations common to all groups living in mountainous regions. Arable bottomland is limited and steep slopes exacerbate erosion on fragile, shallow, upland soils. Recuperation from human or natural perturbations is much slower than in lowland areas. It would be unreasonable to suggest the Cherokee return to traditional subsistence farming practices on worn-out fields or that they should live like their ancestors did and shun the modern world. However, as this chapter demonstrates, there are aspects of the traditional diet that would alleviate some of the contemporary chronic diseases and improve the general health of the population. What was once considered a crude diet for the unrefined is now haute cuisine and relished at inflated prices by health-conscious sophisticates. By reincorporating their traditional foods into their present diet, the Cherokee would be acknowledging their heritage as they improved tribal health conditions.

It would not be difficult to reintroduce or increase the availability of traditional Cherokee foods. Many of the berries mentioned here are now available throughout the year in supermarkets, either as fresh fruit or in the frozen food section. Of course, berries fresh off the bush have better flavor and nutritional profiles. Most of the cultivars of commercially grown berries are from varieties that are native to the southern Appalachian region. Highbush and low-bush blueberries as well as strawberries do quite well on acidic soils as long as there is ample rainfall. Red raspberries are endemic to the high mountains of North Carolina. Elderberries and blackberries are weedy invaders in abandoned fields and fencerows. It would take little effort or expense to assure the Cherokee an ample supply of these fruits, and quality farmland could be used for other purposes. Preservation techniques such as freezing, canning, or drying would extend the season and the benefits.

Nut orchards could be easily established or wild trees managed to increase yields. These would provide a satisfying alternative to current diets high in saturated fats and could be established on any land suitable for deciduous forests. High-quality nut oils are now commercially available and found in the health food sections of many supermarkets.

Reinstating the tradition of the family garden is an excellent way to intensify vegetable production and reintroduce traditional Cherokee foods. The current trend toward identifying with Native American roots would encourage the growing and use of traditional garden crops. If frybread and Indian tacos, relics of government commodity programs, can manifest themselves as traditional Native American foods, it should not be too difficult for educators to reintroduce native dishes and preparation techniques for corn and beans. Also, as an adjunct to gardening, many of the edible wild greens are known garden weeds and take little or no encouragement to assure a plentiful crop.

It is clear from the analysis that many of the current health problems among the Cherokee could be at least partially alleviated through improved dietary practices. Diabetes mellitus, gallstones, and cervical cancer all have strong associations with nutritional imbalances and deficiencies. Incorporation of traditional Cherokee foods can be easily implemented and are some of the best nutritional sources for preventing these diseases and associated complications.

6

# The Sacred Feminine in Cherokee Culture

Healing and Identity

*Jenny James*

> The question of what we think we know about Aboriginal mental health
> is tied to the question of how we think we know it.
> —James B. Waldram, *Revenge of the Windigo*

In a spiritual sense, healing and identity are related. As we heal, we know
more about who we are: we know more about our true self and that our true
self is determined by authentic spiritual needs and fulfillments. A healthy
spiritual identity depends on being healed and living in the processes of
healing. A healed person is a whole person; and a person living in, with, and
through the processes of healing is a person living toward a sound spiritual
identity. When we embrace sacred reality, we are healed by what originates
beyond our control, our scope, and our knowledge. Through that which is
sacred, we reexperience what is sacred within us and the world. We are re-
connected internally and externally.

In the religious language of the Judeo-Christian traditions, spiritual
people live in hope of healing, in faith of overcoming that which is in-
surmountable, and within the transformative love of sacred being, which
changes all things. In the religious language of indigenous traditions, spiritual people live in harmony and balance with all things; in living within the
order of the universe, they reexperience a primal sense of oneness, respect,
and meaning, which likewise is universally transformative. In both religious
orientations, we are restored; we are reconstructed; we are reconciled and
known as who we are, through healing.

## Introduction

Studies of shamanism in Native American and world cultures have typically
given more attention to male shamans, with shamanistic phenomena and
mythic motifs associated with the influence, authority, and power of male

figures (Eliade 1964; Hultkrantz 1997; Larsen 1976; Rogers 1982; Shimony 1989; Vitebsky 1995; Winkelman 1992, 2000).

For example, if one looks at Winkelman 1992, with respect to an emphasis on shamanism as a male activity, one finds that male practitioners of magic, healing, and shamanic arts—within a sexual division of labor model—have high socioeconomic status, political power, moral authority, and contact with gods, and are largely identified as priests and healers engaged in positive acts, while female practitioners do not have status, power, authority, or contact with gods, and are identified, along with some men, as mediums, sorcerers, and witches engaged in marginal or negatives acts (45–46). Since the major activities of the shaman (43) entail healing, protection, divination, food acquisition, agriculture, propitiation, malevolent acts, political/legislative power, property control/taxation, war power, judicial power, and informal political power, and given that Cherokee women and mythic feminine figures have matriarchal influence and autonomy in all these shamanic activities, understanding the place of the sacred feminine in cultural healing and identity is critical for reevaluating the role of women and shamanism in Cherokee culture.

As gender-related issues regarding religion and myth have come to the foreground of Cherokee studies (Albanese 1984; Awiakta 1993; Carney 2005; Churchill 2000; Frost 2000; J. James 1996, 2006; Johnston 2003; McGowan 2006; McLoughlin 1979; Perdue 1998), the question of the role of women in Cherokee culture pre- and post-contact presents methodological challenges to scholars of folklore, religion, and women's studies, as well as to professionals in the medical and mental health fields. The sense of loss of the sacred feminine in Native American traditions is acutely felt inasmuch as matriarchal, matrifocal, and matrilineal cultures were and are negatively impacted by patriarchal conquest. According to McGowan, "Southeastern women have seen their matriarchy destroyed. As women, they once had all the rights and powers that American women today are struggling to obtain, including economic and political power; spiritual equality; the right to proper health care, up to and including abortion on demand; the right to divorce on demand; and the right to call—and call off—war" (2006, 65).

Conquest affected shamanism and religious practices in the past and continues to do so today. Hultkrantz argues that "the impact of Southeastern priest administration and modern acculturation seem to have quenched the original medical spiritualism" (1997, 112). (For a discussion of the Cherokee priestly caste, see Fogelson 1984; Irwin 1992.) In a matriarchal culture, medical spiritualism, the religious experience that supports it, and the knowledge used to practice it must be, in large part, feminine. One wonders, did the Cherokee form a male priestly state in the eighteenth century (Hult-krantz 1997, 106) as an effect of conquest? Were the roles of these priests different from or the same as those of the Cherokee shaman (conjuror)? If males became the main, or sole, interpreters of religion, then would not women's leadership roles in religion, matriarchal structures in shamanism, and a feminine basis for religious experience and practice be negatively altered? Is matriarchal insight needed to bring alive the Cherokee spiritual experience (109), including the "how, why, and when" (112) of Cherokee shamanic practice and the meaning of Cherokee medical formulas?

One must ask, if Cherokee culture is predominantly matriarchal in psychological orientation, matrifocal in cultural meaning, and matrilineal in social power, how are traditional and present-day values affected by the loss of the sacred feminine? Is a matriarchal orientation found in Cherokee shamanism pre- and post-contact? Are healing and identity determined by sacred feminine structures of consciousness in the Cherokee tradition? In short, can Cherokee cultural revitalization, mental health, and tribal identity be significantly strengthened by the reconstruction and recovery of elements of a comprehensive sacred feminine worldview? These are the questions this chapter will begin to address in a systematic manner.

If one starts to sketch analytical patterns of reconstruction and recovery of a matriarchal sensibility and spiritual identity of religious mysteries of the sacred feminine, and of spiritual transformation via feminine structures of consciousness in Native American cultures, such patterns should be developed within the context of specific cultural traditions. As a method of reconstruction and restoration, Eduardo Duran uses an archetypal approach in his clinical practice with indigenous peoples, because depth psychology is spiritually and holistically oriented toward healing, as well as affirmative and supportive of indigenous identity (1984, 2006; Duran and Duran 1995).

Archetypal theory, depth psychology, and psychoanalytic theory are biologically and theologically based, rather than sociologically based, critical approaches. (For general issues of archetypal theory, see Arieti 1956; D. Brown 1970; Drake 1967, 1969; Pratt 1972; Staude 1976; Whitmont 1969. For applications to Native American traditions, see Fleisher, Mudkur, and Reyman 1982.) Archetypal theory presupposes we can understand ethnicity in terms of hermeneutics, not race alone. (See Esonwanne 1992 for a discussion of hermeneutics and race. For discussions of the relation between feminism and Jung's theory of the feminine, see Douglas 1990; Goldenberg 1976;

Lauter and Rupprecht 1985; Strathern 1987; Wehr 1987.) For many scholars, Jung is the great Anglo shaman (see Sandner and Wong 1997; Smyers 2002).

In depth psychology (and archetypal and psychoanalytic theory), cultural retention, change and renewal, and the internal and external factors that affect each are determined by transpersonal and transhistorical paradigms, which structure individual and communal consciousness and experience. As genetic tendencies of the psyche, archetypes are expressed in symbols; are oriented toward values of order, harmony, and balance; and are common to humanity. Because archetypes symbolically resolve spiritual conflicts, the psyche becomes healed, stable, integrated, and whole. Through the symbolic expressions of archetypes in dreams, images, myths, rituals, and cultural life, the individual and community experience mystical transformation, healing of the heart, mind, and body, and identification with nature and all that exists. Through archetypes, healing and identity are cosmologically experienced and known.

Because of its cosmological orientation to spirituality, depth psychology can serve as a bridge between Western approaches (which presuppose a subject/object split) and indigenous approaches (which presuppose holism) to Native American health and wellness (Duran 2006, 5–7). For Duran, historical trauma among indigenous peoples is intergenerational and experienced as a loss of soul, an injury to one's spirit, and a wounding of the individual and collective psyche, as well as the earth. Violence (domestic, social, and historical), oppression (internalized social, historical, and psychological forms), and addictions (such as drugs and alcohol) are inherited disorders that mask anger, anxiety, and depression. The need for healing by indigenous peoples can be met by spiritual therapy and models of healing, such as those found in depth psychology, which take seriously the interconnections between humanity and nature, healer and healed, body and mind/heart.

From his fieldwork with the Ojibwa, Hallowell has concluded that mental health is dependent on values because of the role values play in the integration of the personality. Psychological adjustment is impaired when the personality structure, which emerges from value systems of cultural groups, is ignored. According to Hallowell, acculturation, whether high or low, masks the importance of specific cultural values to psychological health. Personality integration is profoundly impacted by the "unconscious sense of the keen loss of vital central values" in cultural groups. Patterns of overt and covert hostility in interpersonal relations and thwarted maturation processes, which accompany cultural decline, likewise appear in cultures undergoing value change and loss (1972, 592–93). In a relational model, values are key determinants of well-being.

The mythologies of Native peoples, and their root metaphors, like Turtle Island and Howling Coyote, are critical then to indigenous wellness and self-worth because they describe the phenomenological life world of the soul (Duran 2006, 131–37). If the Cherokee tradition is matriarchal in psychological orientation, matrifocal in cultural meaning, and matrilineal in social power, one expects to find strong archetypal feminine figures and root metaphors in Cherokee myth that effect the practice of shamanism and determine cultural values. The manner in which both feminine mythic figures and feminine root metaphors reflect healing and identity should reveal the nature of sacred feminine sensibility and spiritual identity in Cherokee culture, as well as a matriarchal worldview, life world, and psyche.

Scholars of Cherokee culture recognize the strength of sacred feminine power in mythic figures and root metaphors associated with Cherokee shamanism and cultural values (Albanese 1984; Awiakta 1993; Churchill 2000; Fogelson 1980b; Hudson 1984; Irwin 1992; J. James 1996, 2006; Johnston 1993; Perdue 1998). Other considerations—such as the role of women healers, female shamans, and women in religion (Achterberg 1990; Anderson and Young 2004; Allen 1986; Atkinson 1992; Christ 1991; Christ and Plaskow 1992; Cooey, Eakin, and McDaniel 1993; Deusen 2001, 2004; Dixon 1908; Ferguson 1995; Gross 1977; Kidwell 1992; Tedlock 2005), ecofeminism (C. Adams 1993; Diamond and Orenstein 1990; Plant 1989; Ruether 1996), the experience of females in prehistory (Adovasio, Soffer, and Page 2007; Claassen and Joyce 1997), and the nature of cross-cultural motifs associated with women and female deities (Eilberg-Schwartz and Doniger 1995; Weile 1982; Hultkrantz 1986; Sered 1994)—point to a need to examine Cherokee texts for multiple levels of sacred feminine meaning and value.

## Healing

The feminine character of healing and identity in the Cherokee tradition can be accessed through the lens of one shamanic formula, Number 77, from the Swimmer Manuscript. This formula expresses the Archetypal Feminine complex, as found in Cherokee culture, in a condensed but rich form (for an extended discussion of the Archetypal Feminine complex in Cherokee myth, see J. James 2006). Herein we find an ancient female figure, her companion animal, the dog, and her manifestations as corn and the sun.

The Swimmer Manuscript is a collection of medical formulas recorded in Cherokee by the shaman Swimmer, transliterated by Mooney, and edited by Mooney and Olbrechts (1932, 279–81). Mooney describes Cherokee shamanic formulas as "embodying almost the whole of the ancient religion of the Cherokees" (1982, 307). Regarding those formulas shared with him by shamans like Swimmer, Gatiswanasti, Gahuni, Inâli, and Tsiskwa, Mooney says, "The language, the conception, and the execution are all genuinely Indian, and hardly a dozen lines of the hundreds of formulas show a trace of the influence of the white man or his religion. The formulas contained in these manuscripts are not disjointed fragments of a system long since extinct, but are the revelation of a living faith which still has its priests and devoted adherents" (1982, 309).

In Formula 77, a patient with indigestion is cured by a shaman, who calls upon the dogs of the four directions—the Brown dog of "the Sun Land" (south), Black dog of "the Night Land" (west), Blue dog of "the Cold Land" (north), and "two Little Red Dogs, yonder on high, right above" (east)—to remove the offending plant and send down their (curative) saliva. The actions taken by the dogs overcome the distress of the patient, which is caused by an "old Woman," who changes the ingested food plant, making it grow inside the patient's abdomen, thereby causing indigestion.

According to Mooney, the term "old Woman" is a "formulistic name for new corn . . . which . . . originally sprang from the blood of an old woman" (Mooney and Olbrechts 1932, 281). He is referring to the Selu myth in which corn is given to the Cherokee by First Woman through her physical death but metaphysical rebirth as life-sustaining corn. The "old Woman" in the Selu myth overcomes the cosmic imbalance, chaos, and disharmony caused by her murder in giving new life through corn. In contrast, the "old Woman" in Formula 77 of the Swimmer Manuscript *causes* imbalance, chaos, and disharmony. These negative conditions and their manifestation in indigestion must be overcome by the dogs of the four directions, and in particular by the "two Little Red Dogs, yonder on high, right above."

The imbalance, chaos, and disharmony caused by the "old Woman" is "cured" in Formula 77 through the removal of the offending plant and through the saliva of the dogs. Dog saliva has antiseptic qualities. The curing mechanisms of Cherokee Formula 77 parallels Karok shamanism. The Karok of California have female shamans who diagnose illnesses by "crouching" before patients "in a dog-life stance, uttering sounds that resemble the barking of a dog. While doing this, they decipher the cause of the illness and the cure to be used, usually the removal of a disease-causing object" (Rogers 1982, 26–27; see also Maddox 1930, 506–8; Powers 1877, 26).

Hudson describes saliva as a vital principle of life for the Cherokee, subject to pollution and imbalance (1984, 15). As a life force, saliva cures and averts evil (Selare 1939). The two Little Red Dogs are especially interesting insofar as they are located "yonder on high, right above us." The two Little Red Dogs are likely the perihelion, that is, optical phenomena of reflected and refracted light from ice crystals, commonly known as sun spots in science and sun dogs in mythology, which appear on either side of the sun (for an example of sun dogs in myth, see Dorsey 1885). We know from Cherokee myth that the Daughter of the Sun lives "in the middle of the sky, directly above the earth" (Mooney 1982, 252). Her mother, the Sun, stops to visit her each day as she journeys from east to west across the sky vault. The two Little Red Dogs, as mythic figures who appear directly above, invoke the presence of the Sun, a female deity for the Cherokee (Mooney 1982; Swanton 1928), in her noontime manifestation.

The two Little Red Dogs allude then to the Sun. Hudson describes "the most important Cherokee spirit" as both a female grandparent and "the Sun, who was thought to be an old woman. They called her 'grandparent.' She was the source of all warmth and light. Sacred fire was her representative on earth, and for this reason men were supposed to do nothing profane in the presence of sacred fire" (Hudson 1984, 13). Witthoft similarly notes through the testimony of Will West Long (Cherokee informant and authority on Cherokee shamanism) that the domestic hearth fire "was human in thought . . . and was in fact an old woman who was a grandmother in kin terms . . . [and who] would effectively protect the family from witch attack and many other ills" (1983, 72).

The motif of the old woman of the hearth fire is supported by a figure in the Olbrechts/Kilpatrick manuscript on Eastern Cherokee mythology, wherein an old woman is directly likened with fire, inasmuch as she can—through her own power—cook meat as it is held over her head (Kilpatrick and Kilpatrick 1966, 387). Jarvis notes the sacrifice of pieces of meat to the hearth fire (1821, 205–6). Irwin describes an ancient female deity being "strongly associated with the sacred fire of the great seven-sided ceremonial lodge" (1992, 241). Offerings of tobacco are made through fire to the corn mother; fire is also associated with her animal representative, the dog (J. James 1996, 2006). When fire is brought to earth, so too is the Ancient of Days, and the Progenitor of the Cherokee (Payne 1838; J. James 1996, 2006). On earth, fire is the sun's manifestation (Swanton 1928).

In terms of archetypal analysis then, the "old Woman" of Formula 77 is a multivalent, symbolic figure who simultaneously references many feminine figures and levels of meaning, such as the Sun (and the Daughter of the Sun), the sacred Fire, the old Woman of the Hearth, and Corn—the First Woman Ancestor, the Old Woman, and Grandmother—of the Cherokee people (J. James 1996, 2006). A multivalent Archetypal Feminine complex is supported by the testimony of Will West Long, who explains the fire of the hearth and of the square-ground "involved female deities" (Witthoft 1983, 70–71). In view of these many feminine figures and multiple levels of sacred feminine meaning, why would such a figure, who as Corn, Sun, Fire, and Ancestor can positively affect all life, cause imbalance, disorder, and dis-harmony? Why are these negative effects mystically overcome by dog saliva? What is the relation between the woman and dogs in this formula? How does their relationship reflect healing in Cherokee culture? In short, how do the figures of the sacred woman and dog in Formula 77 reflect the sacred feminine sensibility of the Cherokee?

## Identity

Depth psychologist Erich Neumann argues that the Great Mother arche-type is among the first structures of human consciousness (1963, 1995). In the history of consciousness, the Great Mother archetype is the first structure of the conscious self, and as such, she is the first principle deity. It is the Great Mother who has power over birth, life, and death; disease and health; vege-tation and famine; and so forth. Her major animal representative is the dog, who accompanies her, acts on her behalf, and protects her (Neumann 1963; Woloy 1990). Both the Great Mother and the sacred dog archetypes ap-pear in the Payne-Butrick manuscript (the earliest recorded interviews with Cherokee shamans), in Mooney's and Schoolcraft's nineteenth-century col-lections, and on through later Cherokee material in the twentieth century into the 1970s (J. James 1996, 2006). In these texts, the Great Mother and dog archetypes are associated with shamanic, transformative activities. (For an extended discussion of the sacred woman and dog in Cherokee culture, see J. James 1996, 2006.)

The dog is identified with corn, fire, and the sun, and sacred events, that is, the flood, the creation of the Milky Way, and death, in Cherokee my-thology (J. James 1996, 2006). The dog plays a providential role on behalf of the Cherokee in their sacred stories and medical formulas. It is the dog who overcomes rheumatism sent by Little Deer to disrespectful hunters; the dog who saves the Cherokee from the primeval flood; the dog who senses witches and drives them away; the dog who lies upon the hearth, close to the old Woman of the fire; and the dog who creates, through corn, the Milky

Way, the path of the souls to heaven. In all instances, the dog represents the Great Mother archetype. As an archetypal moiety, they are interchangeably identified (J. James 2006). As the Great Mother has religious power and moral authority over all life, so too does the dog. As the Great Mother gives life and health, or disease and death, the dog also heals through canine saliva (again, through antiseptic properties) and sacred power, or, alternatively, the dog bites, kills, and eats that which is dead (J. James 2006; Woloy 1990).

As the representative of the Great Mother, the dog then is interchangeably identified with the "old Woman" and with any of her archetypal forms, such as Corn, Fire, and the Sun, her religious power, and her moral authority. The dog, therefore, can restore a patient with indigestion to wellness in Formula 77. The two Little Red Dogs are located directly above with the Great Mother archetypal figure in Cherokee mythology precisely because they are her companions, protectors, and agents. Because the dogs of the four directions are identified with the Great Mother figures of "old Woman" and Sun in Formula 77, they restore the imbalance, disorder, and disharmony she causes by invoking her positive power (which overcomes her negative action). As the old Woman has power over disease and wellness (Payne 1838; Irwin 1992; J. James 1996, 2006), so too does the dog as her companion animal, her moiety partner, and her representative (J. James 2006). The capacity for transformative healing and the nature of spiritual identity cosmologically shared and created by the Great Mother and dog archetypal pair in Formula 77 are shared and re-created by the patient, the shaman, and the Cherokee in shamanic processes of feminine symbolic healing and spiritual transformation. (For representative discussions of the parameters of symbolic healing in anthropology, see Dow 1986; Moerman 1979. For Jung, Duran, and Cherokee medical spiritualism, healing is a mystical, religious phenomenon.)

## The Sacred Feminine: A Comprehensive Model of Healing and Identity

For Neumann, the Great Mother archetype encompasses all the religious mysteries of transformation during the matriarchal stage of human consciousness, as noted in figure 6.1 (Neumann 1963, 82).

In her positive manifestations, the Great Mother transforms the self through perpetual vegetation mysteries (immortality, rebirth, birth, and fruit) and inspiration mysteries (wisdom, vision, inspiration, and ecstasy). In her negative manifestations, the Great Mother ensnares and devours the self through death mysteries (sickness, extinction, death, and dismember-

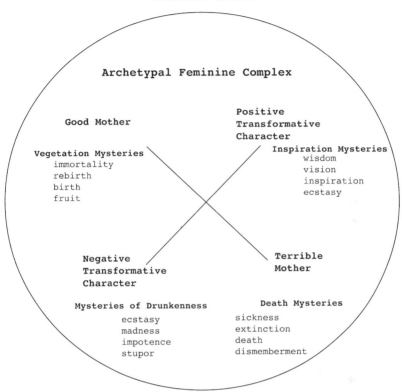

MATRIARCHAL STRUCTURE OF CONSCIOUSNESS
SACRED FEMININE WORLDVIEW
FEMININE LIFE WORLD
FEMININE PSYCHE

Archetypal Feminine Complex

Good Mother

Positive
Transformative
Character

Vegetation Mysteries
  immortality
  rebirth
  birth
  fruit

Inspiration Mysteries
  wisdom
  vision
  inspiration
  ecstasy

Negative
Transformative
Character

Terrible
Mother

Mysteries of Drunkenness
  ecstasy
  madness
  impotence
  stupor

Death Mysteries
  sickness
  extinction
  death
  dismemberment

Figure 6.1. Erich Neumann's Archetypal Feminine complex model. Drawn from Neumann, *The Great Mother: An Analysis of the Archetype*, trans. Ralph Manheim. Bollingen Series XLVII. Princeton: Princeton University Press, 1963.

ment) and through mysteries of drunkenness (ecstasy, madness, impotence, and stupor). The axis of spiritual inspiration—running from both the positive pole of inspiration mysteries to the negative pole of the mysteries of drunkenness—is the root structure of shamanism (Neumann 1963, 64–83). This root structure of matriarchal consciousness defines the feminine motivation of shamanism, that is, to access spiritual life.

Many feminine figures and root metaphors of Cherokee myth express the religious aspects of the Archetypal Feminine complex, that is, the archetypal Good Mother and her perpetual vegetation mysteries of well-being

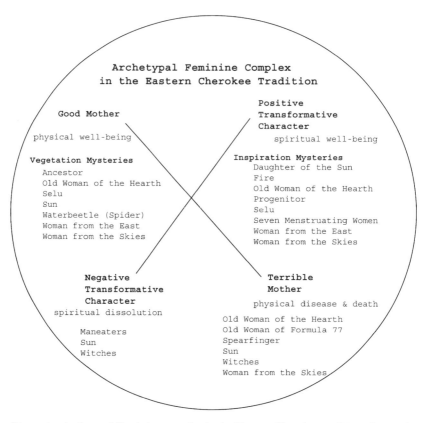

MATRIARCHAL STRUCTURE OF CONSCIOUSNESS
SACRED FEMININE WORLDVIEW
FEMININE LIFE WORLD
FEMININE PSYCHE

Archetypal Feminine Complex
in the Eastern Cherokee Tradition

Good Mother

physical well-being

**Vegetation Mysteries**
 Ancestor
 Old Woman of the Hearth
 Selu
 Sun
 Waterbeetle (Spider)
 Woman from the East
 Woman from the Skies

Positive
Transformative
Character
   spiritual well-being

**Inspiration Mysteries**
 Daughter of the Sun
 Fire
 Old Woman of the Hearth
 Progenitor
 Selu
 Seven Menstruating Women
 Woman from the East
 Woman from the Skies

**Negative
Transformative
Character**
spiritual dissolution

 Maneaters
 Sun
 Witches

**Terrible
Mother**
 physical disease & death

 Old Woman of the Hearth
 Old Woman of Formula 77
 Spearfinger
 Sun
 Witches
 Woman from the Skies

Figure 6.2. Archetypal Feminine complex in the Eastern Cherokee tradition. © 2008 by Jenny James.

and the archetypal Terrible Mother with her death mysteries, as well as the possibility of Psychic Transformation through the positive spiritual mysteries and the possibility of Psychic Dissolution through the negative spiritual mysteries—as seen in figure 6.2.

Significant Cherokee feminine figures and root metaphors are found above at all four poles in this Archetypal Feminine structure of consciousness. For example, in terms of the Good Mother, Selu's religious power and moral authority in vegetation mysteries is well documented in myth (Mooney 1982; Payne 1838) and in ritual, such as the Green Corn Ceremony (Witthoft 1946, 1949). In terms of positive spiritual transformation, the Woman brought down from the skies in the Payne-Butrick manuscript is the cosmogonic earth diver, the origin of life, and the cause of humanity (J. James 1996, 2006). While arguments are made that the Archetypal Great Mother in Native American traditions is exclusively tied to the earth, clearly the Cherokee deity worshiped in the Sun, in the Woman from the East, and in the Woman from the skies is a transcendent sky god, who descends to earth and ascends to the sky at will (J. James 1996, 2006). Never failing to answer those who call upon her for aid, the transcendent feminine archetype in the Cherokee tradition, in all her manifestations, encodes transformative wisdom, vision, inspiration, and ecstasy (see James 1996, 2006).

While sky gods in Indo-European traditions are largely regarded as being male (see E. O. James 1963), the Great Mother archetype is manifest in sky deities. Briffault writes, "The great goddesses owed their existence not to the earth but to their motherhood; and the Great Mother, whether we find her in the ice-fields of the Arctic or the cornfields of Krete, existed before even an ear of corn had been ground in the mill. Her origin was heavenly not earthly, and she had fertilized the dark earth and been the mother of all her fruits long before she was crowned with corn. Hence, however closely Demeter and analogous goddesses may have become assimilated to the Earth-Mother, they could never lose their heavenly character" (1963, 375).

Also at the positive pole of spiritual transformation, are the Seven Menstruating Women, who shamanistically overcome Flint/Stoneclad, a great adversarial figure in Cherokee mythology, through their sacred sexual power (Albanese 1984; Churchill 2000; Fogelson 1980b; Irwin 1992; J. James 1996; Perdue 1998). The nature of sexual power is creativity (Hultkrantz 1997, 164), which cannot be controlled or manipulated by those who do not possess it. The Archetypal Feminine is the elementary, transformative, creative principle, which "encompasses the whole world" (Neumann 1963, 62). As the creative principle of all life, the Archetypal Feminine is one, and its "original unity" is the "highest" expression of "transformation," or "spirit" (Neumann, 1963, 62). The Seven Menstruating Women shamanistically overcome Flint because their power is greater; because their seven persons correspond to the seven levels of spiritual reality in Cherokee metaphysics; and because they carry sacred life itself, with menstruation as their testimony.

The menstruation imagery of the seven women who overcome Flint/Stoneclad is linked to blood, fire, and death (see Albanese 1984). Through the fire they use against him, Flint/Stoneclad dies, and in dying he reveals great secret, sacred cures to the Cherokee people. The blood of Selu is symbolically and religiously linked to the blood of the menstruating women. This blood is also linked to the redness of the Sun and her physical manifestation on earth, fire, and life-giving warmth. Menstruation is a primal sacramental activity that signifies the ultimate shamanic act in matriarchal consciousness, the act of giving life, which is manifest in the transformation of the pregnant female body and the blood of childbirth.

The transformative power of the Seven Menstruating Women cannot be reduced to mere sexuality and/or dialectic of purity and/or pollution because their sacred, creative, transformative power is the life force present in all things, whether fire or corn, life or death, and so forth. Within the Archetypal Feminine complex, the transformation of the female body is metaphoric for the transformation of the human soul. The foundational shamanic realization then is that the soul is changed, healed, or damned by sacred feminine power.

Because they are transformative beings, then, the Seven Menstruating Women defeat Flint/Stoneclad and give magic to the Cherokee people in the form of a beneficial stone (Mooney 1982). The humble Water Spider is another transformative feminine figure in Cherokee myth, who brings fire from the Sun to earth for the Cherokee people in her round tusti bowl. While many other creatures seek fire for the Cherokee and are defeated, the Water Spider is successful because her round bowl is a sacred vessel that symbolizes the same creativity manifested by the Seven Menstruating Women, a capacity she likewise carries within her body. Bowl, or vessel, iconography is part of the Archetypal Feminine complex signifying birth, the female womb, and creativity (see Neumann 1963, 120–46, 211–39).

Sacred feminine creativity is also manifested by the Sun herself, who daily travels across the sky, warming the earth and making it fruitful (Corkran 1955; Hudson 1984; Swanton 1928), and by the old Woman of the Fire, who protects the household and ensures familial well-being (Corkran 1953; Hudson 1984; Witthoft 1983). Each of these sacred feminine mythic figures embodies positive, creative, transformative religious power and moral authority in matrifocal structures of meaning that restore harmony, order, and balance.

The negative death mysteries are found in archetypal feminine figures such as Spearfinger (Mooney 1982), witches (Mooney 1982), and man-eaters (Kilpatrick and Kilpatrick 1966), the Woman from the skies (Payne 1838; J. James 1996, 2006), the old Woman in the fire (J. James 1996, 2006; Witthoft 1983), the old Woman grandparent (Witthoft 1983; Irwin 1992; J. James

1996, 2006; Mooney and Olbrechts 1932), the Sun (Hudson 1984; Irwin 1992; J. James 1996, 2006; Mooney 1982; Swanton 1928), and in Selu (Hudson 1984; Irwin 1992; J. James 1996, 2006; Mooney 1982; Payne 1838), who each cause sickness, disease, and death.

Expressions of the negative mysteries of spiritual dissolution in the Archetypal Feminine complex are found in these feminine figures and root metaphors of Cherokee mythology. The disrespected Fire may cause negative ecstatic experiences, and thus meat offerings and proper caretaking are always given to her (J. James 1996; Jarvis 1821; Witthoft 1983); man-eaters cause ecstatic madness (Kilpatrick and Kilpatrick 1966); the Sun causes madness and death by coming to close to the earth (Irwin 1992; J. James 1996; Mooney 1982); and the Woman from the East (the Woman from the skies, the Sun, and the Grandparent) can turn fertility into infertility and impotence (J. James 1996, 2006; Payne 1838).

The Daughter of the Sun myth illustrates many of the positive and negative manifestations of matriarchal consciousness and structures of the Archetypal Feminine complex found in Cherokee texts. The Daughter of the Sun lives immediately above the Cherokee, occupying the midday position of the sun. Everyday, as the Sun travels from east to west across the sky, the Sun stops at her daughter's house. Since the Sun does not like the Cherokee people, and is jealous of her brother, the Moon, whom the Cherokee like more than her because he does not make them too hot, she intentionally comes too close to the earth in her travels across the sky, and thereby kills them with fever. The Cherokee turn to the Little People for help, and they twice send snakes to kill the Sun. When the snakes fail and unwittingly kill her daughter instead, the Sun mourns, retreats, and leaves the earth in darkness. The Little People then send seven men to bring the Sun's daughter back to her grieving mother in a box from the west, the land of the dead. Almost arriving at the home of the Sun in the east with her captive child, the men relent at the daughter's cries for air and lift the lid of the box, whereupon the Daughter of the Sun escapes as a red bird.

The matriarchal iconography of the Daughter of the Sun myth affirms the Great Mother archetype and the matrifocal life cycles and meaning associated with her on several levels. The Sun, as a Great Mother archetypal figure in Cherokee tradition, has power over life and death, and may take life if she wishes through sickness, that is, fevers or sunstroke. Because of her sacred power, sacred beings, such as the Little People, are consulted. They send sacred snakes (Spreading-adder, Copperhead, Rattlesnake, and Uktena), transformed from men, to kill her. Snakes are the first symbolic manifestation of consciousness and the Great Mother archetype in her first transformative capacity (Neumann 1963, 24–38), which can be manifest—singly or doubly—as life-giving, pregnant Mother and/or devouring Terrible Mother. The sacred snakes, even the mighty Uktena, cannot defeat the Sun because she has power over life and death.

Seven men, with seven being a sacred number in the Cherokee mythos (corresponding to the levels of sacred reality), cannot defeat the Sun's daughter because the Sun, a Great Mother archetype, controls life/death. Her daughter is an extension of herself, and thus her daughter escapes. As an extension of her mother the Sun, the daughter is red (the archetypal color for the sun and fire). As a bird, the daughter is a free soul who flies to her mother. Just as Demeter's Persephone is annually restored to her mother and spring vegetation ensues at her return, so too, when the Daughter of the Sun returns to her mother the Sun, the earth is ultimately renewed. In this story, the Great Mother is doubly present in her first transformation as life giver, the Good Mother, and life taker, the Terrible Mother; she gives life to her daughter and the Cherokee, and gives death to the Cherokee. Psychic transformation is represented in the transformation of the Daughter of the Sun, in the shamanic powers of the Little People, in the men who are transformed into snakes, and in the seven men who represent the seven levels of sacred reality. Psychic dissolution is represented in the actions of the Sun, who will not show herself (and light and warm the earth) when her daughter dies; in the actions of the sacred snakes who twice fail and fall into disarray; and in the action of the seven men, who unthinkingly let the Daughter of the Sun escape.

Given the many sacred feminine figures in figure 6.2, and their presence at each pole of the Archetypal Feminine complex, among the most persistent, exhaustive aspects of sacred reality in the Cherokee tradition is then the sacred feminine. Given the universal power and authority of the feminine figures in Cherokee myth, and the manner in which they balance positive and negative aspects of physical, psychological, and religious/psychic life, if one or all of these forms are unacknowledged, the individual and/or cultural psyche may not be well, whole, and integrated. Given that the foundational concerns of shamanism emerge from these feminine structures in the history of consciousness, that is, from psychic transformation or dissolution, no understanding of healing and identity in any shamanic culture can be complete without them.

The above-described Cherokee feminine figures and root metaphors, which accompany them, express the Archetypal Feminine complex and encode the intentionality of the Cherokee psyche at the matriarchal level of consciousness. The matriarchal structures of consciousness present in Cherokee texts (whether myth or medical formulas) encompass feminine patterns of cultural reconstruction and restoration, and delineate multiple levels of sacred feminine meaning, which are present in the psyche. Fire, Corn, Sun, and Stars are several of the cosmological referents of the Great Mother archetype in Cherokee culture, and these figures and their root metaphors encrypt the nature of feminine sensibility for Cherokee spiritual transformation. These codes describe feminine dimensions of shamanic activities and show us aspects of shamanism other than induced states of altered consciousness and magical flights to other worlds. The Great Mother is present in this world as Corn and Sun, as Fire and protection, and as the reality of life and death, health and sickness, and the Milky Way. The Great Mother archetype is present as positive spiritual transformation or negative spiritual dissolution. Like a mandala, the delineation of the Archetypal Feminine complex in the Cherokee tradition provides a meditative structure for cultural revitalization and psychic healing. Sacred interiority symbolically represented in mandalas may also be replicated in exterior sacred spaces, such as the fire of the seven-sided Cherokee ceremonial lodge (see Irwin 1992), which express group historic identity through complex processes of social order, cultural fusion, and historical development (Albanese 1977).

## A Therapy of Culture

The character of healing in Formula 77 reflects Cherokee matriarchal, matrifocal, and matrilineal identity in a cryptic text. In the Cherokee tradition, psychic transformation is described and encoded within feminine mythic figures such as the Woman from the skies, Selu, the Grandparent, the Sun, the Woman from the East, the old Woman from above, the Daughter of the Sun, the old Woman of the Hearth, Fire, and the Seven Menstruating Women. Root metaphors, that is, the healing dog and protective fire, menacing witches with negative power and menstruating women with sacred sexual power, and the path to the stars being created by the dog and corn, likewise describe and encode psychic transformative power. Through such figures, metaphors, myths, and medical formulas, we perceive Cherokee identity as profoundly feminine and Cherokee healing as a possibility structured by the Archetypal Feminine complex. Without these structures of the sacred feminine, how can one access religious meaning in a matriarchal culture such as Cherokee culture?

Matriarchal structures of consciousness and culture require methods of analysis that include matriarchal meaning and values. Hultkrantz, in his study of shamanism in North American tribes, states, "Among the Cherokee, the idea of spiritual agents of disease is present, but the curing methods (formula recitation, blowing of medicaments, or their infusion) are, except for the ritual moments, devoid of religiously inspired treatment. Knowledge, not visionary experience, directs medical actions" (1997, 160). Again, for Hultkrantz, the epistemological foundation for Cherokee medical spiritualism has been lost.

However, in view of the religious power and moral authority of the Great Mother archetypal complex in Cherokee tradition and the presence of the sacred woman and dog archetypal moiety in Formula 77 of the Swimmer Manuscript, the feminine nature of spiritual reality, vision, religious experience, and knowledge of healing and identity in Cherokee culture was acknowledged at some time in the past, and may provide an epistemological foundation for Cherokee medical spiritualism again, as well as insights into the effects of patriarchy on Cherokee culture post-contact. For example, if the rise of a male priestly caste in eighteenth-century Cherokee culture was influenced by contact with patriarchal Anglo culture, then perhaps the violent struggle between the mother towns and their priestly oppressors (Fogelson 1984) reflects a social struggle between matriarchal loyalists and patriarchal usurpers, and thus represents a conflict of religious identity.

The imagery of the eighteenth-century Cherokee priestly caste is feminine, that is, flowing, long hair, and, according to Fogelson, associated with feminine, sexual images of "night, darkness, and fire." He writes, "Night, of course, is associated with magic and danger, with darkness and the moon, with death and chaos, whereas daytime is related to religious propitiation, to light and the sun, and to life-giving functions and structural order. Fire was considered an earthy equivalent of the sun and was worshipped as a potent deity (Cf. Swanton 1928)" (1984, 259). In Fogelson's description of the images associated with the eighteenth-century Cherokee priestly caste, we see the juxtaposition of the poles of the Archetypal Feminine complex as found in the Cherokee tradition, that is, the Terrible Mother of fire, death, chaos, and the moon (brother and thus matrilineal agent of the feminine sun in the Cherokee tradition) versus the Good Mother of order, sun, life, and light: that is, negative psychic dissolution versus positive psychic transformation as found in the Archetypal Feminine complex (see fig. 6.1).

If the Ani-Kutani (priestly caste) stressed the negative mysteries of death and psychic dissolution (with the positive vegetation and inspiration mysteries being ignored), and distorted and abused feminine sacred sexual power and moral authority, would not the matriarchal Cherokee revolt, as they did, because Cherokee religious identity was being perverted? Was the rise of the Ani-Kutani linked to an eighteenth-century revitalization movement, which distorted the sacred feminine in Cherokee religion? When the Ani-Kutani sang the migration legend, and put out the sacred fire, were they usurping the religious power and moral authority of the sacred feminine for their patriarchal intentions? Were their sexual practices the final apostasy against matriarchal order, harmony, and balance? Did the conflict between a patriarchal revitalization movement in the eighteenth century and a thoroughgoing matriarchal cultural orientation, along with the complexity of acculturation and nineteenth-century removal, confuse and obscure the sacred feminine foundations of medical spiritualism in Cherokee culture? Were some Cherokee shamans (conjurors) pitted against the priestly caste, and left to protect a matriarchal tradition that was in disarray and a matriarchal worldview under assault from within and without? (See Fogelson 1984; Irwin 1992; J. James 1996, 2006.)

Archetypal analysis offers to scholars of folklore, religion, and culture, and to therapists as well, a rich tool that can describe dimensions of healing and identity for particular groups. Fenton argues that methodological considerations of personality structure give the critical historian a technique to approach texts and fieldwork, when direct historical method ends (1948, 514–15). For Goldenberg, archetypes—because they are mystical and ultimately appeal to that which is beyond text—evade patriarchal domination (1976, 449). In addition to providing intentional structures for scholarly and therapeutic examination, archetypes give access into cosmological insights regarding the religious power and moral authority of ancient feminine figures and animals, as well as their cultural roles. The historical trauma model of Duran thus has implications not only for the survival of Native traditions and health but also more broadly for the survival of our planet and all that lives. If our planet is to survive, if cultures and genders are to be revitalized and restored, if animal and plant species are to be retained, healing and identity must involve models and ideologies inclusive of all life forms.

For Neumann, the Western spiritual ethic of perfectionism is eclipsed by depth psychology's spiritual ethic of realism and holism. Violence and psychic disintegration result when one denies weakness, faults, and the shadow self. The moral failure of Western perfectionism in the twentieth, and now the twenty-first, century bears witness to the inability of the West to take responsibility for the repressed darkness of the unconscious mind. When one

acknowledges flaws, insecurities, and ignoble feelings, integration and healing can occur. Such integration and healing is creative and is the "basis for
creative processes which give birth to new values" (Neumann 1990, 101–3).
The archetypal values, which emerge from the unconscious mind into the
conscious cultural canon, will degenerate over time (Neumann 1966, 108–9),
but the genetic impetus and capacity for archetypal expressions will yield
new understandings, values, and canons; that is, new integrations of consciousness.

Morrison describes Hallowell's work on Native American cultural values
as "an understanding of other-than-human persons [that] is foundational
for the study of Native American religious traditions" (2000, 35). He argues
that an interdependent ontology of beings similar to humans is critical for
religious insights into Native American religions. Within such a relational
ontology, that which is sacred cannot be separated from its manifestation or
restricted to a category of being that exists over and against the earth. Perception, behavior, and cognition are intentional, interrelational states of existence shared between human and nonhuman species, with manitou being a shared, intersubjective world (Morrison 2000, 23–54). This quest for
a relational ontology appears in the work of other Native American scholars (Allen 1986; J. Brown 1982, 1997; Harrod 1987, 1995, 2000; Deloria Jr.
1978) and in that of numerous feminist and ecofeminist scholars (Christ and
Plaskow 1992; Cooey, Eakin, and McDaniel 1993; Diamond and Orenstein
1990; Plant 1989; Ruether 1996).

Matriarchal values stress relation, connection, and integration. A structural analysis of the Great Mother archetype, Neumann argues, gives to "the
psychologist of culture" a means of correction to "the one-sidedly patriarchal development of the male intellectual consciousness, which is no longer
kept in balance by the matriarchal world of the psyche. In this sense the ex-
position of the archetypal-psychical world of the Feminine . . . is also a contribution to a future therapy of culture" (1963, xli–xlii). Without the development of a whole, psychological conscience, humanity cannot go forward
(xliii).

The need for psychic balance is a point strongly made by Awiakta in her
work *Selu: Seeking the Corn-Mother's Wisdom* (1993). For Awiakta, respect for
women is a special spiritual gift of the Cherokee that is critical for the health
and well-being of all cultures. The quest for matriarchal understanding can
reconstruct and restore canons of culture in terms of the sacred feminine and
its effect on the psyche. For example, when the universal origin of shamanism is recognized through the Great Mother archetype and a matriarchal

stage of human consciousness, the female attire and mannerisms of male shamans in world cultures (Neumann 1963, 296; Rogers 1982, 26–27; Tedlock 2005, 51) and the influence of the Berdache in Native American traditions (Vitebsky 1995, 93) become explicable.

## Conclusion

The structure of the Archetypal Feminine complex forms a basis for a hermeneutics of the sacred feminine in world religious traditions that is relational, holistic, intersubjective, and inclusive of all forms of life. A hermeneutics of the sacred feminine aids "shamanic revitalization and reconstruction," as described by Tedlock (2005, 270–82), inasmuch as it offers a foundational model that precedes patriarchal consciousness and its effects, that is, a philosophical subject/object split, binary dualisms, racism, sexism, speciesism, and androcentric ethics. One sees through a structural analysis of the Archetypal Feminine complex that the animal mother (Anisimov 1963), the corn mother (Prentice 1986), the Great Mother as the tree of life (Johnson 1994; Neumann 1963), and the Great Mother archetype in all her manifestations are the foundational precursors of shamanic structures, like the world pillar, world tree, and cosmic mountain (Eliade 1987). Through a structural analysis of the Archetypal Feminine complex, we can better understand the ancient imagery of healing, shamanism, and medicine as being feminine in origin (Achterberg 1985, 1990; Tedlock 2005).

The comprehensive influence of matriarchal consciousness in Cherokee culture may be appreciated in a more systematic manner via the Great Mother archetype. Many Cherokee scholars lament the lack of a systematic approach to Cherokee religion and spirituality (Churchill 2000). The sacred power and moral authority of feminine figures and root metaphors in Cherokee myth appear in all four areas of spiritual transformative mysteries of the Great Mother archetype. Thus, it is not surprising that the Cherokee shaman turns to the Woman of the East for rain, to the old Woman of the hearth for blessing and protection, to Selu (the corn mother) for sustenance, and to the Sun for fertility, warmth, and inspiration (J. James 2006), because each is an important religious figure in the Cherokee life world. It is also not surprising that the loss of these cultural symbols and a matriarchal phenomenology would leave one vulnerable to the negative transformative mysteries of drunkenness (ecstasy, madness, impotence, and stupor) and the spiritual vacuums of violence and addiction.

As the primary animal representative of the Great Mother archetype, the dog is identified with her various forms. The shaman invokes the power of the dogs of the four directions in Formula 77 to counter the action taken by the old Woman because the sacred dog can counteract her. That is to say, when the sacred woman is manifest in her negative aspect of sickness and disease, the dog can manifest her positive aspect of healing and wellness. Both the old Woman and the dog encompass an orientation to reality in which life and death, healing and illness, fertility and famine are whole, one, feminine, and sacred. As an archetypal pair, they complement rather than oppose one another, and in so doing point to a holistic approach to Cherokee studies in which comprehensive, rather than dualistic, structures can be described. Mary C. Churchill argues against Hudson's dualistic interpretation of Cherokee tradition and for a holistic, "indigenous-based model of complementarity rather than opposition" (2000, 224–26). Robert K. Thomas also disagrees with Hudson in this matter, feeling Hudson projects a dualism he finds in Creek culture onto Cherokee culture (personal communication).

Symbolic healing, in part, occurs through memory, that is, through its loss and reclamation. After trauma, there is recovery, and the processes of recollection begin when we look for clues about who we are. Considered spiritually, sacred narratives, myths, formulas, and rituals express the healing processes of particular peoples, and how a people come to define themselves as a spiritual group whose true self is known in those symbols, stories, prayers, and rites that celebrate their healing and, out of this healing, celebrate their identity. One symbol, myth, formula, or ritual should, at some level, encode what heals and defines an entire culture and its values. As a pericope, or special text of identity, gives broad insight into many myths and texts, which define biblical peoples, a sacred formula also is a special text of identity. The archetypal structures found therein, in like manner, give broad insight into many myths and texts, which are critical to self-understanding by a cultural group.

In biblical criticism, a pericope is regarded as a short, originally oral, unit of text, which defines an important element of spirituality for a particular people. Other texts and embellishments are added to the pericope, forming larger units of sacred texts. For example, the wandering Aramean speech of Deuteronomy 26:5: "A wandering Aramean was my father; and he went down into Egypt and sojourned there, few in number; and there he became a nation, great, mighty, and populous. And the Egyptians treated us harshly, and afflicted us, and laid upon us hard bondage. Then we cried to the Lord the God of our fathers, and the Lord heard our voice, and saw our affliction, our toil, and our oppression; and the Lord brought us out of Egypt with a mighty hand and an outstretched arm, with great terror, with signs and wonders; and he brought us into this place and gave us this land, a land flowing with milk and honey." Deuteronomy 26:5–9 (RSV) religiously defines the Israelites as that people who are led by God into and out of Egypt and then unto Canaan in order to be saved from their adversaries and to become a great people. Likewise, the kerygma of Mark 1: "Jesus came into Galilee, preaching the gospel of God, and saying "The time is fulfilled, and the Kingdom of God is at hand; repent, and believe in the gospel." Mark 1:14–15 (RSV) defines the first-century Christians as that people who hear the gospel, that is, the kingdom of God is at hand, and repent through Jesus Christ. Additional texts are added to these critical short texts such that, in one sense, the wandering Aramean speech of Deuteronomy 26:5 expresses Jewish identity (and the whole of the Torah and Talmud) in an abbreviated form, as the kerygma of Mark 1 expresses Christian identity (and the whole of the Christian scriptures and tradition) in one slender description.

In the same sense, Formula 77 is a sacred text of medical spiritualism that defines early Cherokees as that people who are healed through the relationship of the sacred woman and dog archetypes. Through the lens of Formula 77, the entire matriarchal life world of the Cherokee may be thus described in a concise way, that is, in this healing archetypal relationship and image, and in these feminine figures and root metaphors of sacred woman and dog, and the greater sacramental, mythological, and textual contexts, which they encompass and encode. (For general insights into the role of the pericope in the analysis of sacred texts, see Anderson 1978. For an application of the pericope concept to other biblical texts, see Willis 1984 on the hearing oracle of the first Isaiah, and Evans 1987 on the true election of the Elijah/Elisha narratives and the "fisher of men" metaphor of Luke.)

An archetypal analysis of Formula 77 from the Swimmer Manuscript demonstrates the religious power and moral authority of the sacred woman and dog archetypes in Cherokee culture in a condensed, culturally encrypted form. These archetypal figures, and their root metaphors of Fire, Flood, Corn, Sky, Soul, and Sun, express the transformative power of the sacred feminine sensibility in Cherokee tradition. They reveal dimensions of what has been retained, and what can be restored and reconstructed in cultural revitalization, in cross-cultural dialogue and in therapeutic settings. The Woman from the skies and the dog in Cherokee myth reflect the sacred figures and root metaphors of Turtle Island and Howling Coyote, cited by Duran. Archetypal analysis shows that which is related ontologically and cosmologically is also related symbolically, and that modes of intersubjective ontological and cosmological being are expressed in modes of intersubjective symbolic being. Together, the Great Mother and dog archetypal moiety in Cherokee culture express a religious worldview and a symbolic cultural canon in which the sacred feminine is foundational, transformative, reconciliatory, and caring (J. James 2006), both in the past and today. They encode a psychic path to healing and identity.

# References

Achterberg, Jeanne. 1985. *Imagery in Healing: Shamanism and Modern Medicine.* Boston: New Science Library.

———. 1990. *Woman as Healer.* Boston: Shambhala Publications.

Acton, Kelly J., Nika Rios Burrows, Kelly Moore, Linda Querec, Linda Geiss, and Michael M. Engelgau. 2002. "Trends in Prevalence among American Indian and Alaska Native Children, Adolescents, and Young Adults." *American Journal of Public Health* 92(9):1485–90.

Adair, James. 1930. *Adair's History of the American Indians.* Johnson City, TN: Watauga Press.

———. 2005. *The History of the American Indians.* Ed. Kathryn Holland Braund. Tuscaloosa: University of Alabama Press.

Adams, Carol J., ed. 1993. *Ecofeminism and the Sacred.* New York: Continuum.

Adams, E. C. 1984. "Archaeology and the Native American: A Case at Hopi." In *Ethics in Archaeology,* ed. E. L. Green, 236–42. New York: The Free Press.

Adhikari, Devi P., Jayaraj A. Francis, Robert E. Schutzki, Amitabh Chandra, and Muraleedharan G. Nair. 2005. "Quantification and Characterization of Cyclooxygenase and Lipid Peroxidation Inhibitory Anthocyanins in Fruits of Amelanchier." *Phytochemical Analysis* 16:175–80.

Adovasio, J. M., Olga Soffer, and Jake Page. 2007. *The Invisible Sex: Uncovering the True Roles of Women in Prehistory.* New York: Smithsonian Books.

Agira, Toshiaki. 2004. "The Antioxidative Function, Preventive Action on Disease, and Utilization of Proanthocyanidins." *BioFactors* 21:197–201.

Ailhaud, Gerard, Florence Massiera, Pierre Weill, Philippe Legrand, Jean-Marc Alessandri, and Philippe Guesnet. 2006. "Temporal Changes in Dietary Fats: Role of n-6 Polyunsaturated Fatty Acids in Excessive Adipose Tissue Development and Relationship to Obesity." *Progress in Lipid Research* 45:203–36.

Albanese, Catherine L. 1977. "The Multi-Dimensional Mandala: A Study in the Interiorization of Sacred Space." *Numen* 24(1):1–25.

———. 1984. "Exploring Regional Religion: A Case Study of the Eastern Cherokee." *History of Religions* 23:344–71.

Allen, Paula Gunn. 1986. *The Sacred Hoop: Recovering the Feminine in American Indian Traditions.* Boston: Beacon Press.

Altman, Heidi M. 2006. *Eastern Cherokee Fishing.* Tuscaloosa: University of Alabama Press.

Anda, Robert F., Janet B. Croft, Vincent J. Felitti, Dale Nordenberg, Wayne H. Giles, David F. Williamson, and Gary A. Giovino. 1999. "Adverse Childhood Experiences and Smoking during Adolescence and Adulthood." *Journal of the American Medical Association* 282(17):1652–58.

Anda, Robert F., Charles L. Whitfield, Vincent J. Felitti, Daniel Chapman, Valerie J. Edwards, Shanta R. Dube, and David F. Williamson. 2002. "Adverse Childhood Experiences, Alcoholic Parents, and Later Risk of Alcoholism and Depression." *Psychiatric Services* 53(8):1001–9.

Andersen, Teri. 1992. "Liver and Gallbladder Disease before and after Very Low-Calorie Diets." *American Journal of Clinical Nutrition* 56:235S–239S.

Anderson, Bernard W. 1978. "From Analysis to Synthesis: The Interpretation of Genesis 1–11." *Journal of Biblical Literature* 97(1):23–39.

Anderson, Leona M., and Pamela Dickey Young. 2004. *Women and Religious Traditions.* Don Mills, Ontario: Oxford University Press.

Anderson, D. C., D. Zieglowsky, and S. Shermer. 1985. *The Study of Ancient Human Skeletal Remains in Iowa: A Symposium.* Iowa City: Office of the State Archeologist of Iowa.

Anisimov, A. F. 1963. "The Shaman's Tent of the Evenks and the Origin of the Shamanistic Rite." In *Studies in Siberian Shamanism,* ed. Henry N. Michael. Toronto: University of Toronto Press.

Anyon, R., and T. J. Ferguson. 1995. "Cultural Resources Management at the Pueblo of Zuni, New Mexico." *Antiquity* 69:919–30.

Anyon, R., and J. Zunie. 1989. "Cooperation at the Pueblo of Zuni: Common Ground for Archaeological and Tribal Concerns." *Practicing Anthropology* 11:13–15.

Arch, Sallie. 2002. "Diabetes Mellitus." *Cherokee One Feather* (Cherokee, NC), August 21, p. 11.

Arieti, Silvano. 1956. "Some Basic Problems Common to Anthropology and Modern Psychiatry." *American Anthropologist,* n.s., 58(1):26–39.

Ariga, Toshiaki. 2004. "The Antioxidative Function, Preventive Action on Disease and Utilization of Proanthocyanidins." *BioFactors* 21:197–201.

Armelagos, G. J., D. S. Carlson, and D. P. Van Gerven. 1982. "The Theoretical Foundations and Development of Skeletal Biology." In *A History of American Physical Anthropology, 1930–1980,* ed. Frank Spencer, 305–29. New York: Academic Press.

Asad, T., ed. 1973. *Anthropology and the Colonial Encounter.* London: Ithaca Press.

Atkinson, Jane Monnig. 1992. "Shamanisms Today." *Annual Review of Anthropology* 21:307–30.

Awiakta, Marilou. 1993. *Selu: Seeking the Corn-Mother's Wisdom.* Golden, CO: Fulcrum Publishing.

Baker, B. J., T. L. Varney, R. G. Wilkinson, L. M. Anderson, and M. A. Liston. 2001. "Repatriation and the Study of Human Remains." In *The Future of the Past: Archaeologists, Native Americans, and Repatriation,* ed. T. L. Bray, 69–89. New York: Garland.

Balzer, Marjorie Mandelstam. 1996. "Flights of the Sacred: Symbolism and Theory in Siberian Shamanism." *American Anthropologist,* n.s., 98(2):305–18.

Bartram, William. 1791. *Travels through North and South Carolina, Georgia, East and West Florida, etc.* Philadelphia: James and Johnson.

Bates, J. F. 1982. "An Analysis of the Aboriginal Ceramic Artifacts from Chota-Tanasee, an Eighteenth-Century Overhill Cherokee Town." M.A. thesis, University of Tennessee, Knoxville.

Beecher, Christopher W. W. 1994. "Cancer Preventive Properties of Varieties of *Brassica Oleracea:* A Review." *American Journal of Clinical Nutrition* 59(supp.):1166S–1170S.

Beekwilder, Jules, Robert D. Hall, and C. H. Ric de Vos. 2005. "Identification and Dietary Relevance of Antioxidants from Raspberry." *BioFactors* 23:197–205.

Begay, D. R. 1991. "Navajo Preservation: The Success of the Navajo Nation Historic Preservation Department." *CRM* 14(1):4.

Begay, R. M. 1997. "The Role of Archaeology on Indian Lands: The Navajo Nation." In *Native Americans and Archaeologists: Stepping Stones to Common Ground,* ed. N. Swidler, K. Dongoske, R. Anyon, and A. Downer, 161–66. Walnut Creek, CA: Alta Mira Press.

Bendich, Adrianne. 1989. "Carotenoids and the Immune Response." *Journal of Nutrition* 119:112–15.

Benyshek, Daniel C. 2001. "The Political Ecology of Diabetes among the Havasupai Indians of Northern Arizona." Ph.D. diss., Arizona State University.

Benyshek, Daniel C., and James T. Watson. 2006. "Exploring the Thrifty Genotype's Food-Shortage Assumptions: A Cross-Cultural Comparison of Ethnographic Accounts of Food Security among Foraging and Agricultural Societies." *American Journal of Physical Anthropology* 131:120–26.

Bever, B. Oliver, and G. R. Zhand. 1979. "Plants with Oral Hypoglycemic Action." *Quarterly Journal of Crude Drug Research* 17(3–4):139–96.

Bieder, R. E. 1990. "A Brief Historical Survey of the Expropriation of American Indian Remains." Manuscript on file at the Native American Rights Fund, Boulder, CO.

———. 1992. "The Collecting of Bones for Anthropological Narratives." *American Indian Culture and Research Journal* 16:21–33.

———. 1996. "The Representations of Indian Bodies in Nineteenth-Century American Anthropology." *American Indian Quarterly* 20:165–79.

Bielawski, E. 1992. "Inuit Indigenous Knowledge and Science in the Arctic." *Northern Perspectives* 20:5–8.

———. 1994. "Dual Perceptions of the Past: Archaeology and Inuit Culture." In *Conflict in the Archaeology of Living Traditions,* ed. R. Layton, 215–22. New York: Routledge.

Bigbee, R. P. 1992. "Anthropometric Variation of the Cherokee, Choctaw, Kiowa and Pawnee Amerindians." M.A. thesis, University of Tennessee.

Bogan, A. E. 1980. "A Comparison of Late Prehistoric Dallas and Overhill Cherokee Subsistence Strategies in the Little Tennessee River Valley." Ph.D. diss., University of Tennessee, Knoxville.

Boik, John. 1996. *Cancer and Natural Medicine: A Textbook of Basic Science and Clinical Research.* Portland: Oregon Medical Press.

Boyce, Vicky L., and Boyd A. Swinburn. 1993. "The Traditional Pima Indian Diet." *Diabetes Care* 16(supp. 1):369–71.

Boyd, T., and J. Haas. 1992. "The Native American Graves Protection and Repatriation Act: Prospects for New Partnerships between Museums and Native American Groups." *Arizona State Law Journal* 24:253–82.

Bray, T. L. 2001. "American Archaeologists and Native Americans: A Relationship under Construction." In *The Future of the Past: Archaeologists, Native Americans, and Repatriation,* ed. T. L. Bray, 1–8. New York: Garland.

Breault, Joseph L. 1997. "A Strategy for Reducing Tuberculosis among Oglala Sioux Native Americans." *American Journal of Preventive Medicine* 13(3): 182–88.

Bressini, Ricardo. 1990. "Chemistry, Technology, and Nutritive Value of Maize Tortillas." *Food Reviews International* 6(2):225–64.

Briffault, Robert. 1963. *The Mothers.* New York: Grosset and Dunlap.

Bright, Mary Anne. 2002. *Holistic Health and Healing.* Philadelphia: F. A. Davis Company.

Brock, K. E., G. Berry, P. A. Mock, R. MacClennan, A. S. Truswell, and L. A. Brinton. 1988. "Nutrients in Diet and Plasma and Risk of In Situ Cervical Cancer." *Journal of the National Cancer Institute* 80(8):580–85.

Broussard, Brenda A., Jonathan R. Sugarman, Karen Bachman-Carter, Karmen Booth, Larry Stephenson, Karen Strauss, and Dorothy Gohdes. 1995. "Toward Comprehensive Obesity Prevention Programs in Native American Communities." *Obesity Research* 3(supp. 2):289S–297S.

Brown, Daniel Russell. 1970. "A Look at Archetypal Criticism." *Journal of Aesthetics and Art Criticism* 28(4):465–72.

Brown, Joseph Epes. 1982. *The Spiritual Legacy of the American Indian.* New York: Crossroad.

——. 1997. *Animals of the Soul: Sacred Animals of the Oglala Sioux.* New York: Element Books.

Brundtland, Gro Harlem. 2002. "Statement from the Director-General of the World Health Organization on World Health Day," April 7, 2002. http://www.who.int/.

Brunner, Eric, and Michael Marmot. 2001. "Social Organization, Stress, and Health." In *Social Determinants of Health,* ed. M. Marmot and R. Wilkinson, 17–43. New York: Oxford University Press.

Brunner, E. J., et al. 2002. "Adrenocortical, Autonomic, and Inflammatory Causes of the Metabolic Syndrome." American Heart Association, Inc. http://www.circulationaha.org/. Pp. 2659–65.

Buikstra, J. 1983. "Reburial: How We All Lose." *Society for California Archaeology Newsletter* 17:1.

Bullock, Ann K. 2001a. "Connection of Stress/Trauma to Diabetes and the Insulin Resistance Syndrome." Unpublished manuscript in possession of the author.

——. 2001b. "Native Americans, Stress, and Type 2 Diabetes: Exploring the Roots of the Epidemic." Unpublished manuscript in possession of the author.

Butterworth, C. E., Kenneth D. Hatch, Maurizio Macaluso, Philip Cole, Howerde E. Sauberlich, Seng-Jaw Soong, Matthew Borst, and Vicki V. Baker. 1992. "Folate Deficiency and Cervical Dysplasia." *Journal of the American Medical Association* 267(4):528–33.

Carney, Virginia Moore. 2005. *Eastern Band Cherokee Women: Cultural Persistence in Their Letters and Speeches.* Knoxville: University of Tennessee Press.

Caroli, A., A. Volpi, and L. Okolicsanyi. 2004. "Gallstone Disease in Diabetics: Prevalence and Associated Factors." *Digestive and Liver Disease* 36:699–700.

Cerdá, B., F. A. Tomás-Barberán, and J. C. Espín. 2005. "Metabolism of Antioxidant and Chemopreventive Ellagitannins from Strawberries, Raspberries,

Walnuts and Oak-Aged Wine in Humans: Identification of Biomarkers and Individual Variability." *Journal of Agricultural Food Chemistry* 53:227–35.

Chapman, J. 1985. *Tellico Archaeology: 12,000 Years of Native American History.* Report of Investigations No. 43. Knoxville: Department of Anthropology, University of Tennessee. Occasional Paper No. 5. Knoxville: Frank H. McClung Museum, University of Tennessee. Publications in Anthropology No. 41. Knoxville: Tennessee Valley Authority, distributed by the University of Tennessee Press.

———. 1988. *The Archaeological Collections at the Frank H. McClung Museum.* Occasional Paper No. 7. Knoxville: Frank H. McClung Museum, University of Tennessee.

———. 1994. *Tellico Archaeology: 12,000 Years of Native American History.* Rev. ed. Knoxville: University of Tennessee Press.

Chapman, Jefferson, Paul A. Delcourt, Patricia A. Cridlebaug, Andrea B. Shea, and Hazel R. Delcourt. 1982. "Man-Land Interaction: 10,000 Years of American Indian Impact on Native Ecosystems in the Lower Little Tennessee River Valley, Eastern Tennessee." *Southeastern Archaeology* 1(2):115–21.

"Cherokee Healing, Reconciliation Day: Working toward Wellness." 2002. *Sylva Herald and Ruralite.* September 19, p. 8A.

Chiltoskey, Mary Ulmer. 1975. "Cherokee Indian Foods." In *Gastronomy: The Anthropology of Food and Food Habits,* ed. Margaret L. Arnott. The Hague: Mouton Press.

Christ, Carol. 1991. "Mircea Eliade and the Feminist Paradigm Shift." *Journal of Feminist Studies of Religion* 7:75–94.

Christ, Carol P., and Judith Plaskow. 1992. *Womanspirit Rising: A Feminist Reader in Religion.* San Francisco: HarperSanFrancisco.

Churchill, Mary C. 2000. "Purity and Pollution: Unearthing an Oppositional Paradigm in the Study of Cherokee Religious Traditions." In *Native American Spirituality: A Critical Reader,* ed. Lee Irwin. Lincoln: University of Nebraska Press.

Claassen, Cheryl, and Rosemary A. Joyce. 1997. *Women in Prehistory: North America and Mesoamerica.* Philadelphia: University of Pennsylvania Press.

Clinton, Steven K. 1998. "Lycopene: Chemistry, Biology, and Implications for Human Health and Disease." *Nutrition Reviews* 56(2):35–51.

Coatsworth, J. H. 1996. "Presidential Address: Welfare." *American Historical Review* 101:1–12.

Cooey, Paula M., William R. Eakin, and Jay B. McDaniel. 1993. *After Patriarchy: Feminist Transformation of the World Religions.* Maryknoll, NY: Orbis Books.

Cooke, Darren, William P. Steward, Andreas J. Gescher, and Tim Marczylo.

2005. "Anthocyans from Fruit and Vegetables—Does Bright Color Signal Cancer Chemopreventive Activity?" *European Journal of Cancer* 41:1931–40.

Corbett, Jane. 1988. "Famine and Household Coping Strategies." *World Development* 16(9):1099–1112.

Cordain, L., J. Miller, and N. Mann. 1999. "Scant Evidence of Periodic Starvation among Hunter-Gatherers." *Diabetologia* 43(3):383–84.

Corkran, David H. 1953. "The Sacred Fire of the Cherokees." *Southern Indian Studies* 5:21–26.

———. 1955. "Cherokee Sun and Fire Observances." *Southern Indian Studies* 8:33–38.

Cozzo, David N. 2004. "Ethnobotanical Classification System and Medical Ethnobotany of the Eastern Band of the Cherokee Indians." Ph.D. diss., University of Georgia, Athens.

Crellin, John K., and Jane Philpott. 1989. *A Reference Guide to Medicinal Plants: Herbal Medicine Past and Present.* Durham: Duke University Press.

Crosby, A. W. 1972. *The Columbian Exchange: Biological and Cultural Consequences of 1492.* Westport, CT: Greenwood.

Defelice, Michael S. 2003. "The Black Nightshades, *Solanum nigrum* et al.— Poison, Poultice, and Pie." *Weed Technology* 17:421–27.

Deloria, Vine, Jr. 1978. *The Metaphysics of Modern Existence.* San Francisco: Harper and Row.

———. 1981. "Identity and Culture." *Daedalus* 110(2):13–27.

Deusen, Kira Van. 2001. *The Flying Tiger: Women Shamans and Storytellers of the Amur.* Montreal: McGill University Press.

———. 2004. *Singing Story, Healing Drum: Shamans and Storytellers of Turkic Siberia.* Seattle: University of Washington Press.

Diamond, Irene, and Gloria Feman Orenstein, eds. 1990. *Reweaving the World: The Emergence of Ecofeminism.* San Francisco: Sierra Club Books.

Dignan, Mark, P. Sharp, K. Blinson, R. Michielutte, J. Konen, R. Bell, and C. Lane. 1994. "Development of a Cervical Cancer Education Program for Native American Women in North Carolina." *Journal of Cancer Education* 9(4):235–42.

Dillinger, Teresa L., Stephen C. Jett, Martha J. Macri, and Louis E. Grivetti. 1999. "Feast or Famine? Supplemental Food Programs and Their Impacts on Two American Indian Communities in California." *International Journal of Food Sciences and Nutrition* 50:173–87.

Dixon, Roland B. 1908. "Some Aspects of the American Shaman." *Journal of American Folklore* 21(80):1–12.

Dobyns, H. F. 1976. *Native American Historical Demography: A Critical Bibliography.* Bloomington: University of Indiana.

———. 1983. *Their Number Become Thinned: Native American Population Dynamics in Eastern North America.* Knoxville: University of Tennessee Press.

Dong, Maxia, Wayne H. Giles, Vincent J. Felitti, Shanta R. Dube, Janice E. Williams, Daniel P. Chapman, and Robert F. Anda. 2004. "Insights into Causal Pathways for Ischemic Heart Disease Adverse Childhood Experiences Study." *Circulation* 110:1761–66.

Dongoske, K. E. 1996. "The Native American Graves Protection and Repatriation Act: A New Beginning, Not the End, for Osteological Analysis—A Hopi Perspective." *American Indian Quarterly* 20:287–96.

Dongoske, K. E., and R. Anyon. 1997. "Federal Archaeology: Tribes, Diatribes, and Tribulations." In *Native Americans and Archaeologists: Stepping Stones to Common Ground,* ed. N. Swidler, K. Dongoske, R. Anyon, and A. Downer, 188–96. Walnut Creek, CA: Alta Mira Press.

Doran, Robert M. 1981. *Psychic Conversion and Theological Foundations: Toward a Reorientation of the Human Sciences.* AAR Studies in Religion 25. Chico, CA: Scholars Press.

Dorsey, J. Owen. 1885. "Siouan Folk-Lore and Mythologic Notes." *American Antiquarian and Oriental Journal* 7(2):105–8.

Douglas, Claire. 1990. *The Woman in the Mirror: Analytical Psychology and the Feminine.* Boston: Sigo Press.

Dow, James. 1986. "Universal Aspects of Symbolic Healing: A Theoretical Synthesis." *American Anthropologist,* n.s., 88(1):56–69.

Drake, Carlos C. 1967. "Jung and His Critics." *Journal of American Folklore* 80(318):321–33.

———. 1969. "Jungian Psychology and Its Uses in Folklore." *Journal of American Folklore* 82(324):122–31.

Drehler, Mark L., Cecelia V. Maher, and Patricia Kearney. 1996. "The Traditional and Emerging Role of Nuts in Healthful Diets." *Nutrition Reviews* 54(8):241–45.

Drewnowski, Adam, and S. E. Specter. 2004. "Poverty and Obesity: The Role of Energy Density and Energy Costs." *American Journal of Clinical Nutrition* 79:6–16.

Dube, Shanta R., Vincent J. Felitti, Maxia Dong, Daniel P. Chapman, Wayne H. Giles, and Robert F. Anda. 2003. "Childhood Abuse, Neglect, and Household Dysfunction and the Risk of Illicit Drug Use: The Adverse Childhood Experiences Study." *Pediatrics* 111(3):564–72.

Duggan, B. J. 1998. "Being Cherokee in a White World: The Ethnic Persistence of a Post-Removal American Indian Enclave." Ph.D. diss., University of Tennessee.

Duke, James A. 1992. *Handbook of Edible Weeds.* Boca Raton: CRC Press.

———. 1997. *The Green Pharmacy: New Discoveries in Herbal Remedies for Common Diseases and Conditions from the World's Foremost Authority on Healing Herbs.* Emmaus, PA: Rodale Press.

Duran, Eduardo. 1984. *Archetypal Consultation: A Service Delivery Model for Native Americans.* New York: Peter Lang.

———. 2002. "Wounding Seeking Wounding: The Psychology of Internalized Oppression." Paper presented at the Healing Our Wounded Spirits Research Conference, May 20, Portland, OR.

———. 2005. "Healing the Soul Wound." Presentation to Health and Medical Division, Eastern Band of Cherokee Indians, July, Cherokee, NC.

———. 2006. *Healing the Soul Wound: Counseling with American Indians and Other Native Peoples.* New York: Teachers College Press.

Duran, Eduardo, and Bonnie Duran. 1995. *Native American Postcolonial Psychology.* Albany: State University of New York Press.

Duran, E., B. Duran, M. Yellow Horse Brave Heart, and S. Yellow Horse-Davis. 1998. "Healing the American Indian Soul Wound." In *International Handbook of Multigenerational Legacies of Trauma,* ed. Yael Danieli, 341–54. New York: Plenum Press.

Eilberg-Schwartz, Howard, and Wendy Doniger, eds. 1995. *Off with Her Head: The Denial of Women's Identity in Myth, Religion, and Culture.* Berkeley: University of California Press.

Eliade, Mircea. 1964. *Shamanism: Archaic Techniques of Ecstasy.* Trans. Willard R. Trask. Bollingen Series LXXVI. Princeton: Princeton University Press.

———. 1987. "Shamanism and Cosmology." In *Shamanism,* ed. Shirley Nicholson. Wheaton, IL: Theosophical Publishing House.

Esonwanne, Uzo. 1992. "'Race' and Hermeneutics: Paradigm Shift—From Scientific to Hermeneutic Understanding of Race." *African American Review* 26(4):565–82.

Evans, Craig A. 1987. "Luke's Use of the Elijah-Elisha Narratives and the Ethic of Election." *Journal of Biblical Literature* 106(1):75–83.

Everhart, James E., Fawn Yeh, Elisa T. Lee, Michael C. Hill, Richard Fabsitz, Barbara V. Howard, and Thomas K. Welty. 2002. "Prevalence of Gallbladder Disease in American Indian Populations: Findings from the Strong Heart Study." *Hepatology* 35(6):1507–12.

Farmer, Deborah F., Ronny A. Bell, and Nancy Stark. 2005. "Cancer Screening among Native Americans in Eastern North Carolina." *Journal of Health Care for the Poor and Underserved* 16:634–42.

Farrell, Mary A., P. A. Quiggins, J. D. Eller, P. A. Owle, K. M. Miner, and E. S. Walkingstick. 1993. "Prevalence of Diabetes and Its Complications in the Eastern Band of the Cherokee Indians." *Diabetes Care* 16(supp. 1):253–56.

Feeley, Ruth M., and Bernice K. Watt. 1970. "Nutritive Values of Foods Distributed under USDA Food Assistance Programs." *Journal of the American Dietetic Association* 57:528–47.

Feeling, Durbin, and William Pulte. 1975. *Cherokee-English Dictionary.* Tahlequah: Cherokee Nation of Oklahoma.

Fenton, William N. 1948. "The Present Status of Anthropology in Northeastern North America: A Review Article." *American Anthropologist,* n.s., 50(3, 1):494–515.

Ferguson, Marianne. 1995. *Women and Religion.* Englewood Cliffs, NJ: Prentice-Hall.

Ferris, Frederick L. 1993. "Diabetic Retinopathy." *Diabetes Care* 16(supp. 1): 322–25.

Feuer, Joshua P. 2001. "Assessment of Acculturation and Its Associations with Type 2 Diabetes, Impaired Glucose Tolerance and Obesity in an Isolated Canadian Aboriginal Community." Master's thesis, University of Toronto.

Finger, J. R. 1984. *The Eastern Band of Cherokees, 1819–1900.* Knoxville: University of Tennessee Press.

———. 1991. *Cherokee Americans: The Eastern Band of Cherokees in the Twentieth Century.* Lincoln: University of Nebraska Press.

Fleisher, Mark Steward, Balaji Mudkur, and Jonathan E. Reyman. 1982. "More on Mandalas, Archetypes, and Native American World Views." *Current Anthropology* 23(3):335–38.

Fogelson, Raymond D. 1958. "A Study of the Conjuror in Eastern Cherokee Society." Master's thesis, University of Pennsylvania.

———. 1961. "Change, Persistence, and Accommodation in Cherokee Medico-Magical Beliefs." In *Symposium on Cherokee and Iroquois Culture,* ed. W. N. Fenton and J. Gulick. Washington, DC: GPO.

———. 1975. "An Analysis of Cherokee Sorcery and Witchcraft." In *Four Centuries of Southern Indians,* ed. Charles M. Hudson. Athens: University of Georgia Press.

———. 1977. "Cherokee Notions of Power." In *The Anthropology of Power: Ethnographic Studies from Asia, Oceania, and the New World,* ed. Raymond D. Fogelson and Richard N. Adams. New York: Academic Press.

———. 1979. "Person, Self, and Identity: Some Anthropological Retrospects, Circumspects, and Prospects." In *Psychosocial Theories of Self,* ed. B. Lee. New York: Plenum Press.

———. 1980a. "The Conjuror in Eastern Cherokee Society." *Journal of Cherokee Studies* 5(2):60–87.

———. 1980b. "Windigo Goes South: Stoneclad among the Cherokees." In *Man-*

*like Monsters on Trial: Early Records and Modern Evidence,* ed. Marjorie M. Halpin and Michael M. Ames. Vancouver: University of British Columbia Press.

———. 1983. "Who Were the Ana-Kuani? An Excursion into Cherokee Historical Thought." *Ethnohistory* 4:255–63.

———. 1985. "Interpretations of the American Indian Psyche: Some Historical Notes." In *Social Contexts of American Ethnology, 1840–1984,* ed. June Helm. Washington, DC: American Ethnological Society.

Fogelson, Raymond D., and Amelia B. Walker. 1980. "Self and Other in Cherokee Booger Masks." *Journal of Cherokee Studies* 5(2):88–101.

———. 1983. "Cherokee Booger Mask Tradition." In *The Power of Symbols: Masks and Masquerade in the Americas,* ed. N. Ross Crumrine and Marjorie Halpin. Vancouver: University of British Columbia Press.

Foreman, Grant. 1932. *Indian Removal.* Norman: University of Oklahoma Press.

Frost, Julieanna. 2000. "Folklore and Female Gender: A Comparative Study of the Cherokee and Creek Nations." Master's thesis, Eastern Michigan University.

Gahagan, Sheila, and Janet Silverstein. 2003. "Committee on Native American Child Health and Section on Endocrinology." *Pediatrics* 112:e328.

Gardner, Paul S. 1997. "The Ecological Structure and Behavioral Implications of Mast Exploitation Strategies." In *People, Plants, and Landscapes: Studies in Paleoethnobotany,* ed. K. J. Gremillion, 161–78. Tuscaloosa: University of Alabama Press.

Garza, C. E., and S. Powell. 2001. "Ethics and the Past: Reburial and Repatriation in American Archaeology." In *The Future of the Past: Archaeologists, Native Americans, and Repatriation,* ed. T. L. Bray, 37–56. New York: Garland.

Giegerich, Wolfgang. 1975. "Ontogeny = Phylogeny? A Fundamental Critique of Erich Neumann's Analytical Psychology." In *Carl Gustav Jung: Critical Assessments,* ed. Renos K. Papadopoulos, 138–54. New York: Routledge.

Gillen, Lynda J., Linda C. Tapsell, Craig C. Patch, Alice Owen, and Marijka Batterham. 2005. "Structured Dietary Advice Incorporating Walnuts Achieves Optimal Fat and Energy Balance in Patients with Type 2 Diabetes Mellitus." *Journal of the American Dietetic Association* 105(7):1087–96.

Gillum, Richard Frank, Brenda S. Gillum, and Norine Smith. 1984. "Cardiovascular Risk Factors among Urban American Indians: Blood Pressure, Serum Lipids, Smoking, Diabetes, Health Knowledge, and Behavior." *Progress in Cardiology* 107(4):765–76.

Giuliano, Anna R. 2000. "The Role of Nutrients in the Prevention of Cervical Dysplasia and Cancer." *Nutrition* 16(7–8):570–73.

Gohdes, Dorothy, Stephen Kaufman, and Sarah Valway. 1993. "Diabetes in American Indians." *Diabetes Care* 16(supp. 1):239–43.

Goldenberg, Naomi R. 1976. "A Feminist Critique of Jung." *Signs* 2(2):443–49.

Goldstein, L., and K. Kintigh. 1990. "Ethics and the Reburial Controversy." *American Antiquity* 55:585–91.

Goodman, Elizabeth, and Robert Whitaker. 2002. "A Prospective Study of the Role of Depression in the Development and Persistence of Adolescent Obesity." *Pediatrics* 109(3):497–504.

Goodwin, Gary C. 1977. "Cherokees in Transition: A Study of Changing Culture and Environment Prior to 1775." University of Chicago Department of Geography Research Paper No. 181.

Greene, L. K. 1996. "The Archaeology and History of the Cherokee Out Towns." Master's thesis, University of Tennessee.

Grim, John A. 2000. "Cultural Identity, Authenticity, and Community Survival: The Politics of Recognition in the Study of Native American Religions." In *Native American Spirituality: A Critical Reader*, ed. Lee Irwin. Lincoln: University of Nebraska Press.

Grimes, R. L. 2001. "Desecration: An Inter-religious Controversy." In *The Future of the Past: Archaeologists, Native Americans, and Repatriation*, ed. T. L. Bray, 91–105. New York: Garland.

Grivetti, Louis E., and Britta M. Ogle. 2000. "Value of Traditional Foods in Meeting Macro- and Micronutrient Needs: The Wild Plant Connection." *Nutrition Research Reviews* 13:31–46.

Gross, Rita M. 1977. *Beyond Androcentrism: New Essays on Women and Religion*. Missoula, MT: Scholars Press.

Hallowell, A. Irving. 1972. "Values, Acculturation and Mental Health." In *The Emergent Native Americans: A Reader in Culture Contact*, ed. Deward E. Walker Jr. Boston: Little, Brown.

Hamilton, M. D. 1999. "Oral Pathology at Averbuch (40DV60): Implications for Health Status." Master's thesis, University of Tennessee.

Handler, R. 1991. "Who Owns the Past? History, Cultural Property, and the Logic of Possessive Individualism." In *The Politics of Culture*, ed. B. Williams, 63–74. Washington, DC: Smithsonian Institution Press.

Hanley, Anthony J. G., Stewart B. Harris, Joel Gittleson, Thomas M. S. Wolever, Brit Saksvig, and Bernard Zinman. 2000. "Overweight among Children and Adolescents in a Native Canadian Community: Prevalence and Associated Factors." *American Journal of Clinical Nutrition* 71:693–700.

Harjo, Susan Shown. 1989. "Indian Remains Deserve Respect." *San Jose Mercury News*, October 10.

———. 2005. "Harjo: My New Year's Resolution: No More Fat 'Indian' Food."

Indian Country Today, January 20. http://www.indiancountry.com/content. cfm?id=1096410209 (site no longer accessible).

Harrod, Howard L. 1984. "Missionary Life-World and Native Response: Jesuits in New France." *Studies in Religion* 13:2.

———. 1987. *Renewing the World: Plains Indian Religion and Morality.* Tucson: University of Arizona Press.

———. 1995. *Becoming and Remaining a People: Native American Religions on the Northern Plains.* Tucson: University of Arizona Press.

———. 2000. *The Animals Came Dancing: Native American Sacred Ecology and Animal Kinship.* Tucson: University of Arizona Press.

Hatley, Thomas. 1991. "Cherokee Women Farmers Hold Their Ground." In *Appalachian Frontiers: Settlements, Society, and Development in the Preindustrial Era,* ed. R. D. Mitchell, 37–51. Lexington: University Press of Kentucky.

Heaps, W. A. 1970. *Riots, U.S.A.* New York: Seabury Press.

Heaton, K. W. 1984. "The Role of Diet in the Aetiology of Cholelithiasis." *Nutrition Abstract Reviews* 54(7):551–60.

Helman, Cecil G. 1994. *Culture, Health, and Illness: An Introduction for Health Professionals.* 3rd ed. Boston: Butterworth-Heinemann.

Herrero, Rolando, Nancy Potischman, Louise A. Brinton, William C. Reeves, Maria M. Brenes, Francisco Tenorio, Rosa C. de Britton, and Eduardo Gaitan. 1991. "A Case-Control Study of Nutrient Status and Invasive Cervical Cancer." *American Journal of Epidemiology* 134(11):1335–55.

Higginbotham, D. 1982. "Native Americans versus Archaeologists: The Legal Issues." *American Indian Law Review* 10:91–115.

Hiss, Blythe. 2008. "Introduction." http://www.ncpad.org/disability/fact_sheet. php?sheet=324&section=1983.

Hjemdahl, P. 2002. "Stress and the Metabolic Syndrome, American Heart Association, Inc." http://www.circulationaha.org/. Pp. 2634–36.

Ho, Gloria Y. F., P. R. Palan, J. Basu, S. Romney, A. S. Kadish, M. Mikhail, S. Wassertheil-Smoller, C. Runowicz, and R. D. Burk. 1998. "Viral Characteristics of Human Papillomavirus Infection and Antioxidant Levels as Risk Factors for Cervical Dysplasia." *International Journal of Cancer* 78:594–99.

Hotu, S., B. Carter, P. D. Watson, W. S. Cutfield, and T. Cundy. 2004. "Increasing Prevalence of Type 2 Diabetes in Adolescence." *Journal of Pediatric Child Health* 40:201–4.

Howard, A. E. 1997. "An Intrasite Spatial Analysis of Surface Collections at Chattooga (38OC18): A Lower Town Cherokee Village." Master's thesis, University of Tennessee.

Hoxie, F. E. 1985. "The Indians versus the Textbooks: Is There Any Way Out?" *AHA Perspectives* 23:18–22.

Hubert, J. 1994. "A Proper Place for the Dead: A Critical Review of the 'Reburial' Issue." In *Conflict in the Archaeology of Living Traditions,* ed. R. Layton, 131–66. New York: Routledge.

Hudson, Charles. 1984. *Elements of Southeastern Indian Religion.* Leiden: E. J. Brill.

Hughes, L. H. 1982. "Cherokee Death Customs." Master's thesis, University of Tennessee.

Hultkrantz, Åke. 1986. "The Religion of the Goddess in North America." In *The Book of the Goddess: Past and Present,* ed. Carl Olson. New York: Crossroad.

———. 1997. *Shamanic Healing and Ritual Drama: Health and Medicine in Native North American Religious Traditions.* New York: Crossroad.

Humphrey, D. C. 1973. "Dissection and Discrimination: The Social Origins of Cadavers in America, 1760–1915." *Bulletin of the New York Academy of Medicine* 49:819–27.

Huttlinger, K. W. 1995. "A Navajo Perspective of Diabetes." *Community Health* 18:9–16.

Irwin, Lee. 1992. "Cherokee Healing: Myth, Dreams, and Medicine." *American Indian Quarterly* 17(2):237–57.

Jackson, P. E. 1950. *The Law of Cadavers and of Burials and Burial Places.* New York: Prentice-Hall.

James, Jenny. 1996. "A Reconstructive Hermeneutic of Eastern Cherokee Spirituality via the Theology of Bernard Lonergan." Ph.D. diss., Toronto: University of St. Michael's College.

———. 2006. "The Dog Tribe." *Southern Anthropologist* 32(1/2):17–46.

James, E. O. 1963. *The Worship of the Sky-God: A Comparative Study in Semitic and Indo-European Religion.* London: Athlone.

Jang, Young P., Jilin Zhou, Koji Nakanishi, and Janet R. Sparrow. 2005. "Anthocyanins Protect against A2E Photooxidation and Membrane Permeabilization in Retinal Pigment Epithelial Cells." *Photochemistry and Photobiology* 81:529–36.

Jarvis, Samuel Farmar. 1821. "A Discourse of the Religion of the Indian Tribes of North America." *Collections of the New-York Historical Society.* Vol. 3.

Jayaprakasam, Bolleddula, Shaiju K. Vareed, L. Karl Olson, and Muraleedharan G. Nair. 2005. "Insulin Secretion by Bioactive Anthocyanins and Anthocyanidins Present in Fruits." *Journal of Agricultural and Food Chemistry* 53(1):28–31.

Joe, J. R., and R. S. Young, eds. 1994. *Diabetes as a Disease of Civilization: The Impact of Culture Change on Indigenous Peoples.* New York: Mouton de Gruyter.

Johnson, Buffie. 1994. *Lady of the Beasts: The Great Mother and Her Sacred Animals.* Rochester, VT: Inner Traditions International.

Johnston, Carolyn Ross. 2003. *Cherokee Women in Crisis: Trail of Tears, Civil War, and Allotment, 1838–1907.* Tuscaloosa: University of Alabama Press.

Jones, Leon D. 2003. "Principal Chief Leon D. Jones' Speech to Tribal Members, Thursday, August 26." *Cherokee One Feather.* August 27, p. 8.

Kalt, Wilhelmina, Charles F. Forney, Antonio Martino, and Ronald L. Prior. 1999. "Antioxidant Capacity, Vitamin C, Phenolics, and Anthocyanins after Fresh Storage of Small Fruits." *Journal of Agricultural and Food Chemistry* 47(11):4638–44.

Kalt, Wilhelmina, Daniel A. J. Ryan, Joanna C. Duy, Ronald L. Prior, Mark K. Ehlenfeldt, and S. P. Vander Kloet. 2001. "Interspecific Variation in Anthocyanins, Phenolics, and Antioxidant Capacity among Genotypes of Highbush and Lowbush Blueberries (*Vaccinium* Section *cyanococcus* spp.)." *Journal of Agricultural and Food Chemistry* 49(10):4761–67.

Karapanagiotidis, Ioannis T., Michael V. Bell, David C. Little, Amararatne Yakupittyage, and Sudip K. Rakshit. 2006. "Polyunsaturated Fatty Acid Content of Wild and Farmed Talapias in Thailand: Effects of Aquaculture Practices and Implications for Human Nutrition." *Journal of Agricultural and Food Chemistry* 54:4304–10.

Katz, Solomon H., N. L. Hediger, and L. A. Valleroy. 1975. "Traditional Maize Processing Techniques in the New World." *Science* 184:765–73.

Katzenberg, M. A., and S. R. Saunders, eds. 2000. *Biological Anthropology of the Human Skeleton.* New York: Wiley-Liss.

Keel, Bennie. 2007. "The Ravensford Tract Archaeological Project." Tallahassee, FL: Southeast Archaeological Center.

Kehoe, Alice Beck. 2000. *Shamans and Religion: An Anthropological Exploration in Critical Thinking.* Prospect Heights, IL: Waveland Press.

Key, Timothy. 1994. "Micronutrients and Cancer Aetiology: The Epidemiological Evidence." *Proceedings of the Nutrition Society* 53:605–14.

Kidwell, Clara Sue. 1992. "Indian Women as Cultural Mediators." *Ethnohistory* 39(2):97–107.

Kilpatrick, Alan. 1997. *The Night Has a Naked Soul: Witchcraft and Sorcery among the Western Cherokee.* Syracuse: Syracuse University Press.

Kilpatrick, Jack Frederick, and Anna Gritts Kilpatrick. 1965. *Walk in Your Soul: Love Incantations of the Oklahoma Cherokees.* Dallas: Southern Methodist University Press.

———. 1966. *Eastern Cherokee Folktales: Reconstructed from the Field Notes of Frans M. Olbrechts.* Smithsonian Institution, Bureau of American Ethnology Bulletin 196. Washington, DC: GPO.

———. 1967. *Run toward the Nightland: Magic of the Oklahoma Cherokees.* Dallas: Southern Methodist University Press.

———. 1970. *Notebook of a Cherokee Shaman.* Washington, DC: Smithsonian Institution Press.

Kim, Young-In. 1999. "Folate and Cancer Prevention: A New Medical Application of Folate beyond Hyperhomocysteinemia and Neural Tube Defects." *Nutrition Reviews* 57(10):314–21.

King, Duane H. 1983. *The Cherokee Indian Nation: A Troubled History.* Knoxville: University of Tennessee Press.

Klein, Laura F., and Lillian A. Ackerman, eds. 1995. *Women and Power in Native North America.* Norman: University of Oklahoma Press.

Klesert, A. L. 1992. "A View from Navajoland on the Reconciliation of Anthropologists and Native Americans." *Human Organization* 51:17–22.

Klesert, A. L., and M. J. Andrews. 1988. "The Treatment of Human Remains on Navajo Lands." *American Antiquity* 53:310–20.

Klesert, A. L., and A. S. Downer, eds. 1990. "Preservation on the Reservation: Native Americans, Native American Lands and Archaeology." Navajo Nation Papers in Anthropology No. 26. Windowrock, AZ: Navajo Nation Archaeology Department and the Navajo Nation Historic Preservation Department.

Koehler, Lyle. 1982. "Native Women of the Americas: A Bibliography." *Frontiers* 6(1):73–101.

Koss, M. 2005. "Adverse Childhood Exposures and Alcohol Dependence among Seven Native American Tribes." *American Journal of Preventive Medicine* 25(3):238–44.

Kroll, Jerome. 2003. "Posttraumatic Symptoms and the Complexity of Responses to Trauma." *Journal of the American Medical Association* 290(5):667–70.

Kupferer, Harriet Jane. 1966. *The "Principal People," 1960: A Study of Cultural and Social Groups of the Eastern Cherokee.* Smithsonian Institution. Anthropological Papers No. 78. Bureau of American Ethnology Bulletin 196. Pp. 215–325. Washington, DC: GPO.

Landau, P. M., and D. G. Steele. 1996. "Why Anthropologists Study Human Remains." *American Indian Quarterly* 20:209–28.

Larsen, C. S. 1982. "The Anthropology of St. Catherine's Island No. 3: Prehistoric Human Biological Adaptation." *Anthropological Papers of the American Museum of Natural History* 57:159–207.

Larsen, Stephen. 1976. *The Shaman's Doorway: Opening the Mythic Imagination to Contemporary Consciousness.* New York: Harper and Row.

Lauter, Estella, and Carol Schreier Rupprecht. 1985. *Feminist Archetypal Theory: Interdisciplinary Re-visions of Jungian Thought.* Knoxville: University of Tennessee Press.

Lefler, Lisa J. 1996. "Mentorship as an Intervention Strategy in Relapse Reduction among Native American Youth." Ph.D. diss., University of Tennessee.

———. 2001. "Issues in Alcohol-Related Problems among Southeastern Indians: Anthropological Approaches." In *Anthropologists and Indians in the New South,* ed. R. A. Bonney and J. A. Paredes, 89–107. Tuscaloosa: University of Alabama Press.

Lewis, Thomas M., and Madeline Kneberg. 1958. *Tribes That Slumber: Indians of the Tennessee Region.* Knoxville: University of Tennessee Press.

Liburd, Leandris C., Leonard Jack, Sheree Williams, and Pattie Tucker. 2005. "Intervening on the Social Determinants of Cardiovascular Disease and Diabetes." *American Journal of Preventive Medicine* 29(5):18–24.

Liu, Zhijun, Joshua Schwimer, Dong Liu, Frank L. Greenway, Catherine T. Anthony, and Eugene A. Woltering. 2005. "Black Raspberry Extract and Fractions Contain Angiogenesis Inhibitor." *Journal of Agricultural and Food Chemistry* 53(10):3909–15.

Loe, Harold. 1993. "Periodontal Disease." *Diabetes Care* 16(supp. 1):329–34.

Loomis, D., and S. Wing. 1990. "Is Molecular Epidemiology a Germ Theory for the End of the Twentieth Century?" *International Journal of Epidemiology* 19:1–3.

Lopez-Ridaura, Ruy, Walter C. Willett, Eric B. Rimm, Simin Liu, Meir J. Stampfer, JoAnn E. Manson, and Frank B. Hu. 2004. "Magnesium Intake and Risk of Type 2 Diabetes in Men and Women." *Diabetes Care* 27(1): 134–40.

Lowe, Lynn P., D. Tranel, R. B. Wallace, and T. K. Welty. 1994. "Type 2 Diabetes and Cognitive Function." *Diabetes Care* 17(8):891–96.

Lunenfeld, M. 1991. *1492: Discovery, Invasion, Encounter.* Lexington, MA: D.C. Heath and Company.

Lurie, N. O. 1988. "Relations between Indians and Anthropologists." In *Handbook of North American Indians,* vol. 4, *History of Indian-White Relations,* ed. W. Washburn, 548–56. Washington, DC: Smithsonian Institution Press.

"Lycopene." 2003. *Alternative Medicine Review* 8(3):336–42.

Lyon, William S. 2004. "Divination in North American Indian Shamanic Healing." In *Divination and Healing: Potent Vision,* ed. Michael Winkelman and Philip M. Peek. Tucson: University of Arizona Press.

Maclure, K. Malcolm, K. C. Hayes, G. A. Colditz, M. J. Stampfer, F. E. Speizer, and W. C. Willett. 1988. "Weight, Diet, and the Risk of Symptomatic Gallstones in Middle-aged Women." *New England Journal of Medicine* 321(9):563–69.

Maddox, John Lee. 1930. "The Spirit Theory in Early Medicine." *American Anthropologist,* n.s., 32(1):503–21.

Maltz, Daniel, and JoAllyn Archambault. 1995. "Gender and Power in Native North America." In *Women and Power in Native North America,* ed. Laura F. Klein and Lillian A. Ackerman. Norman: University of Oklahoma Press.

Manson, S., J. Beals, T. O'Nell, J. Piasecki, D. Bechtold, E. Keane, M. Jones. 1998. "Wounded Spirits, Ailing Hearts: PTSD and Related Disorders among American Indians." In *Ethnocultural Aspects of Posttraumatic Stress Disorder,* ed. Anthony J. Marsella et al., 255–84. Washington, DC: American Psychological Association.

Marmot, Michael, and Richard G. Wilkinson, eds. 2001. *Social Determinants of Health.* New York: Oxford University Press.

Martin-Hill, Dawn. 2004. "Women in Indigenous Traditions." *Women and Religious Traditions,* ed. Leona M. Anderson and Pamela Dickey Young. Don Mills, Ontario: Oxford University Press.

Martin, R. 1997. "How Traditional Navajos View Historic Preservation: A Question of Interpretation." In *Native Americans and Archaeologists: Stepping Stones to Common Ground,* ed. N. Swidler, K. Dongoske, R. Anyon, and A. Downer, 128–34. Walnut Creek, CA: Alta Mira Press.

Mascio, Paolo, Stephan Kaiser, and Helmut Sies. 1989. "Lycopene as the Most Efficient Biological Carotenoid Singlet Oxygen Quencher." *Archives of Biochemistry and Biophysics* 274(1):532–38.

McCarty, Mark F. 2005. "Magnesium May Mediate the Favorable Impact of Whole Grains on Insulin Sensitivity by Acting as a Mild Calcium Antagonist." *Medical Hypothesis* 64:619–27.

McDermott, Robyn. 1999. "Ethics, Epidemiology, and the Thrifty Gene: Biological Determinism as a Health Hazard." *Social Science and Medicine* 47(9): 1189–95.

McDowell, William L., Jr. 1958. *Colonial Records of South Carolina, Documents Relating to Indian Affairs, May 21, 1750–August 7, 1754.* Columbia: South Carolina Archives Department.

McEwen, Bruce, with Elizabeth N. Lasley. 2002. *The End of Stress As We Know It.* Washington, DC: Joseph Henry Press.

McGowan, Kay Givens. 2006. "Weeping for the Lost Matriarchy." In *Daughters of Mother Earth: The Wisdom of Native American Women,* ed. Barbara Alice Mann. Westport, CT: Praeger.

McLoughlin, William G. 1979. "Cherokee Anomie, 1794–1809: New Roles for Red Men, Red Women, and Black Slaves." In *Uprooted Americans,* ed. Richard L. Bushman, Boston: Little, Brown.

———. 1986. *Cherokee Renascence in the New Republic.* Princeton: Princeton University Press.

McLoughlin, William G., and Walter H. Conser Jr. 1977. "The Cherokees in Transition: A Statistical Analysis of the Federal Cherokee Census of 1835." *Journal of American History* 64:678–703.

McMahon, Sarah K., Aveni Haynes, Nirubasini Ratnam, Maree T. Grant,

Christine L. Carne, Timothy Jones, and Elizabeth A. Davis. 2004. "Increase in Type 2 Diabetes in Children and Adolescents in Western Australia." *Medical Journal of Australia* 180:495–61.

McMichael, Anthony J. 1999. "Globalization and the Sustainability of Human Health: An Ecological Perspective." *BioScience* 49(3):205–10.

Mendez-Sanchez, Narhum, Norberto C. Chavez-Tapia, Daniel Motola-Kuba, Karla Sanchez-Lara, Guadalupe Ponciano-Rodriguez, Hector Baptista, Martha H. Ramos, and Misael Uribe. 2005. "Metabolic Syndrome as a Risk Factor for Gallstone Disease." *World Journal of Gastroenterology* 11(11): 1653–57.

Messer, Lynne, Allan Steckler, and Mark Dignan. 1999. "Early Detection of Cervical Cancer among Native American Women: A Qualitative Supplement to a Quantitative Study." *Health Education and Behavior* 26(4):547–62.

Messina, Mark J. 1999. "Legumes and Soybeans: Overview of Their Nutritional Profiles and Health Effects." *American Journal of Clinical Nutrition* 70(supp.):439S–450S.

Mihesuah, D. 2000. "American Indians, Anthropologists, Pothunters, and Repatriation: Ethical, Religious, and Political Differences." In *Repatriation Reader: Who Owns American Indian Remains?* ed. D. Mihesuah, 95–105. Lincoln: University of Nebraska Press.

Millet, S., K. DeCenlaer, W. van Paemal, K. Raes, S. De Smet, and G.P.J. Janssens. 2006. "Lipid Profiles in Eggs of Araucana Hens Compared with Lohmann Selected Leghorn and ISA Brown Hens Given Diets with Different Fat Sources." *British Journal of Poultry Science* 47(3):294–300.

Mitscherlich, A., and F. Mielke. 1947. *Doctors of Infamy: The Story of the Nazi Medical Crimes.* New York: Schuman.

Moerman, Daniel E. 1979. "Anthropology of Symbolic Healing." *Current Anthropology* 20(1):59–80.

———. 2003. *Native American Ethnobotany: A Database of Foods, Drugs, Dyes and Fibers of Native American Peoples, Derived from Plants.* http://herb.umd.umich.edu/.

Mohan, V. 2004. "Why Are Indians More Prone to Diabetes?" *Journal of the Association of Physicians of India* 52:468–74.

Mooney, James. 1890. "Cherokee Theory and Practice of Medicine." *Journal of American Folklore* 3(8):44–50.

———. [1891, 1900] 1992. *History, Myths, and Sacred Formulas of the Cherokees: Containing the Full Texts of Myths of the Cherokee.* Fairview, NC: Bright Mountain Books.

———. 1982. *Myths of the Cherokees and Sacred Formulas of the Cherokees.* Nashville: Charles and Randy Elder Booksellers.

Mooney, James, and Frans M. Olbrechts. 1932. *The Swimmer Manuscript: Cherokee Sacred Formulas and Medicinal Prescriptions.* Smithsonian Institution, Bureau of American Ethnology Bulletin 99. Washington, DC: U.S. GPO.

Moreno, L. A., and G. Rodríguez. 2007. "Dietary Risk Factors for Development of Childhood Obesity." *Current Opinion in Clinical Nutrition and Metabolic Care* 10(3):336–41.

Morrison, Kenneth M. 2000. "The Cosmos as Intersubjective: Native American Other-Than-Human Persons." In *Indigenous Religions: A Companion,* ed. Graham Harvey. New York: Cassell.

Morton, S. G. 1848. *Account of a Craniological Collection.* Transcripts of the American Ethnological Society II. New York.

Mozaffarian, Dariush, Martijn B. Katan, Alberto Ascherio, Meir J. Stampfer, and Walter C. Willitt. 2006. "Trans Fatty Acids and Cardiovascular Disease." *New England Journal of Medicine* 354:1601–13.

Mukherjee, Pulok K., Kuntal Maiti, Kakali Mikherjee, and Peter J. Houghton. 2006. "Leads from Indian Medicinal Plants with Hypoglycemic Potentials." *Journal of Ethnopharmacology* 106:1–28.

Mullen, William, Jennifer McGinn, Michael E. Lean, Margaret R. MacLean, Peter Gardner, Garry G. Duthie, Takoa Yokota, and Alan Crozier. 2002. "Ellagitannins, Flavonoids, and Other Phenolics in Red Raspberries and Their Antioxidant Capacity and Vasorelaxation Properties." *Journal of Agricultural and Food Chemistry* 50(18):5191–96.

Nakeeb, Attila, Anthony G. Comuzzie, Hayder Al-Azzawi, Gabriele E. Sonnenberg, Ahmed H. Kissebah, and Henry A. Pitt. 2002. "Insulin Resistance Causes Human Gallbladder Dysmotility." *Journal of Gastrointestinal Surgery* 10(7):940–49.

Narayan, K. M. Venkat. 1996. "Diabetes Mellitus in Native Americans: The Problem and Its Implications." In *Changing Numbers, Changing Needs: American Indian Demography and Public Health,* ed. G. D. Sandefur, R. R. Rindfuss, and B. Cohen. Washington, DC: National Academy Press.

Neely, Sharlotte. 1979. "Acculturation and Persistence among North Carolina's Eastern Band of the Cherokee." In *Southeastern Indians since the Removal Era,* ed. W. L. Williams, 154–73. Athens: University of Georgia Press.

Nelkin, D., and L. Andrews. 1998. "Do the Dead Have Interests? Policy Issues for Research after Life." *American Journal of Law and Medicine* 24:261–91.

Nervi, Flavo, C. Covarrubias, P. Bravo, N. Velasco, N. Ulloa, F. Cruz, M. Fava, C. Severin, R. Del Pozo, C. Antezana, V. Valdivieso, and A. Arteaga. 1989. "Influence of Legume Intake on Biliary Lipids and Cholesterol Saturation in Young Chilean Men." *Gastroenterology* 96:825–30.

Neumann, Erich. 1963. *The Great Mother: An Analysis of the Archetype.* Trans.

Ralph Manheim. Bollingen Series XLVII. Princeton: Princeton University Press.

———. 1966. *Art and the Creative Unconscious.* New York: Harper Torchbooks.

———. 1990. *Depth Psychology and a New Ethic.* New York: Shambala.

———. 1994. *The Fear of the Feminine and Other Essays on Feminine Psychology.* Princeton: Princeton University Press.

———. 1995. *The Origins and History of Consciousness.* Bollingen Series XLII. Princeton: Princeton University Press.

Newmark, Harold L. 1996. "Plant Phenolics as Potential Cancer Prevention Agents." In *Dietary Phytochemicals in Cancer Prevention and Treatment,* 25–34. American Institute for Cancer Research. New York: Plenum Press.

Nott, J. C. 1855. "Types of Mankind: Or, Ethnological Researches, Based Upon the Ancient Monuments, Paintings, Sculptures, and Crania of Races, and Upon Their Natural, Geographical, Philological and Biblical History: Illustrated by Selections from the Unedited Papers of Samuel George Morton . . . and by Additional Contributions from Prof. L. Agassiz, LL.D., W. Usher, M.D., and Prof. H. S. Patterson, M.D. By J. C. Nott and Geo. R. Gliddon." Philadelphia: Lippincott Gramoo and Company.

Odegaard, Andrew O., and Mark A. Pereira. 2006. "Trans Fatty Acids, Insulin Resistance, and Type 2 Diabetes." *Nutrition Reviews* 64(8):364–72.

Okuda, Takuo, Takashi Yoshida, and Tsutomu Hatano. 1988. "Ellagitannins as Active Constituents of Medicinal Plants." *Planta Medica* 55(2):117–22.

Olson, Brooke. 2001. "Meeting the Challenges of American Indian Diabetes: Anthropological Perspectives on Prevention and Treatment." In *Medicine Ways: Disease, Health, and Survival among Native Americans,* ed. Clifford E. Trafzer and Diane Weiner, 163–84. Walnut Creek, CA: Alta Mira Press.

Olson, James Allan. 1989. "Biological Action of Carotenoids." *Journal of Nutrition* 119:94–95.

Owsley, D. W., and D. T. Bellande. 1982. "Culturally Induced Dental Alterations in a Historic Cherokee Sample." *Journal of Cherokee Studies* 7:82–84.

Owsley, D. W., and B. L. Guevin. 1982. "Cranial Deformation—A Cultural Practice of the Eighteenth Century Overhill Cherokee." *Journal of Cherokee Studies* 7:79–81.

Owsley, D. W., and H. L. O'Brien. 1982. "Stature of Adult Cherokee Indians during the Eighteenth Century." *Journal of Cherokee Studies* 7:74–78.

Paredes, J. Anthony. 1992. "Federal Recognition and the Poarch Creek Indians." In *Indians of the Southeastern United States in the Late 20th Century,* ed. J. Anthony Paredes, 120–22. Tuscaloosa: University of Alabama Press.

Parker, G. Keith. 2006. *Seven Cherokee Myths.* Jefferson, NC: McFarland.

Payne, John Howard. 1838. *Payne-Butrick Manuscript* #689. Vols. 1–14 (in collaboration with D. S. Butrick). Edward E. Ayer and Frank C. Deering Collection, Newberry Library, Chicago.

Pearce, N. 1996. "Traditional Epidemiology, Modern Epidemiology, and Public Health." *American Journal of Public Health* 86:678–83.

Pengelly, Andrew. 1997. *The Constituents of Medicinal Plants: An Introduction to the Chemistry and Therapeutics of Herbal Medicines.* Stanley Cottage: Sunflower Herbals.

Perdue, Theda. 1998. *Cherokee Women: Gender and Culture Change, 1700–1835.* Lincoln: University of Nebraska Press.

Perdue, T., and M. D. Green. 1995. *The Cherokee Removal: A Brief History with Documents.* New York: St. Martin's Press.

Perry, Bruce D., and Maia Szalavitz. 2006. *The Boy Who Was Raised as a Dog: What Traumatized Children Can Teach Us about Loss, Love, and Healing.* New York: Basic Books.

Perry, Myra Jean. 1974. "Food Use of 'Wild' Plants by Cherokee Indians." Master's thesis, University of Tennessee.

Plant, Judith, ed. 1989. *Healing the Wounds: the Promise of Ecofeminism.* Toronto: Between the Lines.

Polhemus, R. 1987. *The Toqua Site: A Late Mississippian Dallas Phase Town.* Report of Investigations No. 41. Knoxville: Department of Anthropology, University of Tennessee.

Potischman, Nancy. 1993. "Nutritional Epidemiology of Cervical Neoplasia." *Journal of Nutrition* 123:424–29.

Pouwer, F., G. Nijpels, A. T. Beekman, J. M. Dekker, R. M. van Dam, R. J. Heine, and F. J. Snoek. 2005. "Fat Food for a Bad Mood: Could We Treat and Prevent Depression in Type 2 Diabetes by Means of ω-3 Polyunsaturated Fatty Acids? A Review of the Evidence." *Diabetic Medicine* 22:1465–75.

Powell, M. L. 1988. *Status and Health in Prehistory.* Washington, DC: Smithsonian Institution Press.

Powers, Stephen. 1877. *Tribes of California.* Contributions to North American Ethnology III. Washington, DC: GPO.

Pratt, Vernon. 1972. "Biological Classification." *British Journal for the Philosophy of Science* 23(4):305–27.

Prentice, Guy. 1986. "An Analysis of the Symbolism Expressed by the Birger Figurine." *American Antiquity* 51(2):239–66.

Prior, Ronald L., Guohua Cao, Antonio Martin, Emin Sofic, John McEwen, Christine O'Brien, Neal Lischner, Mark Ehlenfeldt, Willy Kalt, Gerard Krewer, and C. Mike Mainland. 1998. "Antioxidant Capacity as Influenced by Total Phenolic and Anthocyanin Content, Maturity, and Variety of *Vaccinium* Species." *Journal of Agricultural Food Chemistry* 46:2686–93.

Quiggins, Patricia Ann. 1990. "Insulin Dependent (Type II) Diabetes Mellitus in the Eastern Cherokee of Western North Carolina." Ph.D. diss., University of Tennessee.

Quiggins, Patricia A., and Mary Anne Farrell. 1993. "Renal Disease among the Eastern Band of Cherokee Indians." *Diabetes Care* 16(supp. 1):342–45.

Quintin, Ellison, and Jon Ostendorff. 2002. "Churches to Offer Apology to Cherokees." *Asheville Citizen-Times,* July 21.

Rajaram, Sujatha, and Joan Sabate. 2006. "Nuts, Body Weight, and Insulin Resistance." *British Journal of Nutrition* 96(supp. 2):S79-S-86.

Rajyalakshmi, K., K. Venkatalaxmi, K. Kenkatalakshamamma, Y. Joythsna, K. Balachandramani Devi, and V. Suneetha. 2001. "Total Carotenoid and Beta-Carotene Contents of Forest Green Leafy Vegetables Consumed by Tribals of South India." *Plant Foods for Human Nutrition* 56:225–38.

Reeves, William C., William E. Rawls, and Louise A. Brinton. 1989. "Epidemiology of Genital Papillomaviruses and Cervical Cancer." *Review of Infectious Diseases* 11(3):426–39.

Reinhard, Karl L., and Naomi I. Greenwalt. 1975. "Epidemiological Definition of the Cohort of Diseases Associated with Diabetes in Southwestern American Indians." *Medical Care* 13(2):160–73.

Richardson, R. 1987. *Death, Dissection, and the Destitute.* London: Routledge and Kegan Paul.

Rieder, Hans L. 1989. "Tuberculosis among American Indians of the Contiguous United States." *Public Health Reports* 104(6):653–57.

Riggs, Brett H. 1999. "Removal Period Cherokee Households in Southwestern North Carolina: Material Perspectives on Ethnicity and Cultural Differentiation." Ph.D. diss., University of Tennessee.

———. 2002. "In Service of Native Interests: Archaeology for, of, and by Cherokee People." In *Southern Indians and Anthropologists,* ed. Lisa J. Lefler and Frederic W. Gleach, 19–30. Southern Anthropological Society No. 35. Athens: University of Georgia Press.

Riserus, Ulf. 2006. "*Trans* Fatty Acids and Insulin Resistance." *Atherosclerosis Supplements* 7:37–39.

Ritenbaugh, Cheryl, and Carol Sue Goodby. 1989. "Beyond the Thrifty Gene: Metabolic Implications of Prehistoric Migration into the New World." *Medical Anthropology* 11:227–36.

Roberfroid, Marcel B. 1999. "Concepts on Functional Foods: The Case of Inulin and Oligofructose." *Journal of Nutrition* 129:1398S–1401S.

Roberfroid, M. B., and N. M. Delzenne. 1998. "Dietary Fructans." *Annual Review of Nutrition* 18:117–43.

Robertson, Laurel, Carol Flinders, and Brian Ruppenthal. 1986. *The New Laurel's Kitchen.* Berkeley: Ten Speed Press.

Rodning, C. B. 2001. "Mortuary Ritual and Gender Ideology in Protohistoric

Southwestern North Carolina." In *Archaeological Studies of Gender in the Southeastern United States,* ed. J. M. Eastman and C. B. Rodning, 77–100. Gainesville: University Press of Florida.

Roemer, Kenneth M. 1994. "Contemporary American Indian Literature: The Centrality of Canons on the Margins." *American Literary History* 6:3:583–99.

Rogers, Spencer L. 1982. *The Shaman: His Symbols and His Healing Power.* Springfield, IL: Charles C. Thomas Publisher.

Rose, J. C., J. C. Green, and V. D. Green. 1996. "NAGPRA IS FOREVER: Osteology and the Repatriation of Skeletons." *Annual Review of Anthropology* 25:81–103.

Rotberg, R. I., and T. K. Rabb. 1985. *Hunger and History: The Impact of Changing Food Production and Consumption Patterns on Society.* Cambridge: Cambridge University Press.

Ruether, Rosemary Radford. 1996. *Women Healing Earth: Third World Women on Ecology, Feminism, and Religion.* Marynoll, NY: Orbis Books.

Rumessen, Juri Johannes, Susan Bode, Ole Hamberg, and Eivind Gudmand-Hoyer. 1990. "Fructans of Jerusalem Artichokes: Intestinal Transport, Absorption, Fermentation, and Influence on Blood Glucose Insulin, and C-Peptide Responses in Healthy Subjects." *Journal of Clinical Nutrition* 52: 675–81.

Salare, R. 1939. "A Collection of Saliva Superstitions." *Folklore* 50(4):349–66.

"*Sambucus nigra*" (Elderberry). 2005. *Alternative Medicine Review* 10(1):51–55.

Samuels, Andrew. 1985. *Jung and the Post-Jungians.* Boston: Routledge and Kegan Paul.

Sandner, Donald F., and Steven H. Wong. 1997. *The Sacred Heritage: The Influence of Shamanism on Analytical Psychology.* New York: Routledge.

Sapolsky, Robert. 1998. *Why Zebras Don't Get Ulcers.* New York: W. H. Freeman.

———. 2003. "Taming Stress." *Scientific American.* September, pp. 87–95.

Sattlet, Richard A. 1995. "Women's Status among the Muskogee and Cherokee." In *Women and Power in Native North America,* ed. Laura F. Klein and Lillian A. Ackerman. Norman: University of Oklahoma Press.

Saunders, S. R., and M. A. Katzenberg, eds. 1992. *Skeletal Biology of Past Peoples: Research Methods.* New York: Wiley-Liss.

Sawday, J. 1995. *The Body Emblazoned: Dissection and the Human Body in Renaissance Culture.* London: Routledge.

Scalzo, Jessica, Bruno Mezzetti, and Maruizio Battino. 2005. "Total Antioxidant Capacity Evaluation: Critical Steps for Assaying Berry Antioxidant Features." *BioFactors* 23:221–27.

Schrag, B. 2002. "With Bones in Contention: Repatriation of Human Remains." Commentary. Online Ethics Center for Engineering and Science, Case Western Reserve University. http://onlineethics.org/CMS/5158. aspx?SearchTerm=With+Bones+in+Contention (accessed December 2007).

Schroedl, G. F. 1986a. *Overhill Cherokee Archaeology at Chota-Tanasee.* Report of Investigations No. 38. Knoxville: Department of Anthropology, University of Tennessee.

———. 1986b. *Overhill Cherokee Archaeology at Chota-Tanasee.* N.p.: TVA Publications in Anthropology No. 42.

Schultz, Leslie O., Peter H. Bennett, Eric Ravussin, Judith R. Kidd, Kenneth K. Kidd, Julian Esparza, and Mauro E. Valencia. 2006. "Effects of Traditional and Western Environments on a Prevalence of Type 2 Diabetes in Pima Indians in Mexico and the U.S." *Diabetes Care* 29(8):1866–71.

"Scientific Research and the Autonomy of Indigenous Peoples: The Case of the Kennewick Man." Commentary. 2002. Online Ethics Center for Engineering and Science at Case Western Reserve University. http://onlineethics. org/CMS/research/rescases/gradres/gradresv2/kennewick.aspx (accessed December 2007).

Segura, Ramon, Casimiro Javierre, M. Antonia Lizarraga, and Emilio Ros. 2006. "Other Relevant Components of Nuts: Phytosterols, Folate, and Minerals." *British Journal of Nutrition* 96(supp. 2):S36–S44.

Sellappan, Subramani, Casimir C. Akoh, and Gerard Krewer. 2002. "Phenolic Compounds and Antioxidant Capacity of Georgia-Grown Blueberries and Blackberries." *Journal of Agricultural and Food Chemistry* 50(8):2432–38.

Sellers, Elizabeth, A. C. 2000. "The Emerging Epidemic of Type 2 Diabetes Mellitus in First Nation Children and Youth: Issues Related to Diagnosis, Etiology, Complications and Treatment." Master's thesis. Winnipeg: University of Manitoba.

Sered, Susan Starr. 1994. *Priestess, Mother, Sacred Sister: Religions Dominated by Women.* New York: Oxford University Press.

Shaheb, Sudah. 1990. "Cholelithiasis among American Indians." *Gastroenterology* 98(1):251–52.

Shamdasani, Sonu. 2003. *Jung and the Making of Modern Psychology: The Dream of a Science.* New York: Cambridge University Press.

Shimony, Annemarie. 1985. "Iroquois Religion and Women in Historical Perspective." In *Women, Religion, and Social Change,* ed. Yvonne Yazbeck Hadda and Ellison Banks Findly. Albany: State University of New York Press.

———. 1989. "Eastern Woodlands: Iroquois of Six Nations." In *Witchcraft and Sorcery of the American Native Peoples,* ed. Deward E. Walker Jr. Moscow: University of Idaho Press.

Shonkoff, Jack P., and Deborah A. Phillips, eds. 2000. *From Neurons to Neighborhoods: The Science of Early Childhood Development.* National Research

Council and Institute of Medicine. Washington, DC: National Academy Press.

Sievers, Maurice L., and Jeffery R. Fisher. 1981. "Diseases of North American Indians." In *Biocultural Aspects of Disease,* ed. H. Rothschild. New York: Academic Press.

Simopoulos, A. P. 2006. "Evolutionary Aspects of Diet, the Omega-6/Omega-3 Ratio and Genetic Variation: Nutritional Implications for Chronic Disease." *Biomedicine & Pharmacotherapy* 60:502–7.

Smith, Janell, and Dennis Wiedman. 2001. "Fat Content of South Florida Indian Frybread: Health Implications for a Pervasive Native-American Food." *Journal of the American Dietetic Association* 101(5):582–85.

Smith, M. T. 1987. *Archaeology of Aboriginal Culture Change in the Interior Southeast: Depopulation during the Early Historic Period.* Gainesville: University of Florida Press.

Smyers, Karen A. 2002. "Shaman/Scientist: Jungian Insights for the Anthropological Study of Religion." *Ethos* 29(4):475–90.

Snipp, C. Matthew. 1996. "The Size and Distribution of the American Indian Population: Fertility, Mortality, and Migration." In *Changing Numbers, Changing Needs: American Indian Demography and Public Health,* ed. G. D. Sandefur, R. R. Rindfuss, and B. Cohen. Washington, DC: National Academy Press.

Sockbeson, H. J. 1994. "The Larsen Bay Repatriation Case and Common Errors of Anthropologists." In *Reckoning with the Dead: The Larsen Bay Repatriation and the Smithsonian Institution,* ed. T. L. Bray and T. W. Killion, 158–62. Washington, DC: Smithsonian Institution Press.

Speakman, J. R. 2006. "Thrifty Genes for Obesity and the Metabolic Syndrome— Time to Call off the Search?" *Diabetes & Vascular Research* 3(1):7–11.

Starkloff, Carl F. 1974. *The People of the Center: American Indian Religion and Christianity.* New York: Seabury Press.

Staude, John Raphael. 1976. "From Depth Psychology to Depth Sociology: Freud, Jung, and Levi-Strauss." *Theory and Society* 3(3):303–38.

Steckel, R. H. 1993. "Stature and the Standard of Living." Paper presented at the conference A History of Health and Nutrition in the Western Hemisphere, Ohio State University, Columbus.

Steckel, R. H., and J. C. Rose, eds. 2003. *The Backbone of History: Health and Nutrition in the Western Hemisphere.* Oxford: Cambridge University Press.

Stein, Jay, Kelly M. West, James M. Robey, Dean F. Tirador, and Glen McDonald. 1965. "The High Prevalence of Abnormal Glucose Tolerance in the Cherokee Indians of North Carolina." *Archives of Internal Medicine* 16(December):842–45.

Stivers, Deann Lee. 1990. "Changes in Stature and Health Status as Related to the Emergence of Diabetes among Eastern Cherokee Indians in North Carolina." Ph.D. diss., University of Tennessee.

St.-Onge, Marie-Pierre, Kathleen L. Keller, and Steven B. Heymsfield. 2003. "Changes in Childhood Food Consumption Patterns: A Cause for Concern in Light of Increasing Body Weight." *American Journal of Clinical Nutrition* 78:1068–73.

Story, Mary. 1980. "Food and Nutrient Intake Practices, and Anthropometric Data of Cherokee Indian High School Students in Cherokee, North Carolina." Ph.D. diss., Florida State University.

Story, Mary, Mary Ann Bass, and Lucille M. Wakefield. 1985. "Use of Traditional Indian Foods by Cherokee Youths in Cherokee, North Carolina." *Journal of the American Dietetic Association* 85(8):975–77.

Storey, R. 1992. *Life and Death in the Ancient City of Teotihuacán: A Modern Paleodemographic Synthesis.* Tuscaloosa: University of Alabama Press.

Strathern, Marilyn. 1987. "An Awkward Relationship: The Case of Feminism and Anthropology." *Journal of Women in Culture and Society* 12(2):276–92.

Stroehla, Berrit C., Lorraine Halinka Malcoe, and Ellen M. Velie. 2005. "Dietary Sources of Nutrients among Rural Native American and White Children." *Journal of the American Dietetic Association* 105(12):1908–16.

Sullivan, L. P. 1987. "The Mouse Creek Phase Household." *Southeastern Archaeology* 6:16–29.

Sullivan, L. P., and S. C. Prezzano, eds. 2001. *Archaeology of the Appalachian Highlands.* Knoxville: University of Tennessee Press.

Swanton, John R. 1928. "Sun Worship in the Southeast." *American Anthropologist,* n.s., 30:206–13.

Szathmary, E. J. E. 1986. "Diabetes in Arctic and Subarctic Populations Undergoing Acculturation." *Collegium Anthropologicum* 10:145–58.

Tapsell, Linda C., Lynda J. Gillen, Craig S. Patch, Marijka Batterham, Alice Owen, Marian Bare, and Meredith Kennedy. 2004. "Including Walnuts in a Low-Fat/Modified-Fat Diet Improves HDL Cholesterol-to-Total Cholesterol Ratios in Patients with Type 2 Diabetes." *Diabetes Care* 27(12):2777–83.

Taussig, M. T. 1987. *Shamanism, Colonialism and the Wild Man.* Chicago: University of Chicago Press.

Tedlock, Barbara. 2005. *The Woman in the Shaman's Body: Reclaiming the Feminine in Religion and Medicine.* New York: Bantam Books.

Teltow, Glenna J., James D. Irvin, and Gary M. Aron. 1983. "Inhibition of Herpes Simplex Virus DNA Synthesis by Pokeweed Antiviral Protein." *Antimicrobial Agents and Chemotherapy* 23(3):390–96.

Terry, Rhonda Dale. 1982. "Diet, Anthropometric Characteristics, and Diabetes-

Related Attitudes and Knowledge among Women Residing in the Eastern Cherokee Township of Snowbird." Ph.D. diss., University of Tennessee.

Thomas, Clayton L., ed. 1997. *Taber's Cylcopedic Medical Dictionary.* Philadelphia: F. A. Davis Company.

Thomas, D. H. 2000. *Skull Wars: Archaeology and the Search for Native American Identity.* New York: Basic Books.

Thornton, Russell. 1987. *American Indian Holocaust and Survival: A Population History since 1492.* Norman: University of Oklahoma Press.

———. 1990. *The Cherokees: A Population History.* Lincoln: University of Nebraska Press.

Timberlake, Lieut. Henry. 1765. *Memoirs of Lieut. Henry Timberlake.* London.

Townsend, R. G., and M. H. Hamilton. 2004. "Prehistoric Skeletal Studies: Benefits to Modern Cherokee Communities." Paper presented at the 27th Annual Appalachian Studies Conference. March 27. Cherokee, NC.

Trafazer, Clifford E., and Diane Weiner, eds. 2001. *Medicine Ways: Disease, Health, and Survival among Native Americans.* Walnut Creek, CA: Alta Mira Press.

Tran, Khoi Q., Matthew I. Goldblatt, Deborah A. Swartz-Basile, Carol Svatek, Atilla Nakeeb, and Henry A. Pitt. 2003. "Diabetes and Hyperlipidemia Correlates with Gallbladder Contractility in Leptin-Related Murine Obesity." *Journal of Gastrointestinal Surgery* 7(7):857–63.

Trigger, B. 1980. "Archaeology and the Image of the American Indian." *American Antiquity* 45:662–76.

Trosper, Ronald L. 1996. "American Indian Poverty on Reservations, 1969–1989." In *Changing Numbers, Changing Needs: American Indian Demography and Public Health,* ed. G. D. Sandefur, R. R. Rindfuss, and B. Cohen. Washington, DC: National Academy Press.

Trujillo, Michael H. 2000. "One Prescription for Eliminating Health Disparity—Legislation." *Indian Health Service Fact Sheet.* January.

Tsai, Chung-Jyi, Michael F. Leitzmann, Walter C. Willett, and Edward L. Giovannucci. 2004a. "A Prospective Cohort Study of Nut Consumption and the Risk of Gallstone Disease in Men." *American Journal of Epidemiology* 160(10):961–68.

———. 2004b. "Frequent Nut Consumption and Decreased Risk of Cholecystectomy in Women." *American Journal of Clinical Nutrition* 80:76–81.

———. 2005. "Long Term Intake of Trans-Fatty Acids and Risk of Gallstone Disease in Men." *Archives of Internal Medicine* 165:1011–15.

———. 2006. "Fruit and Vegetable Consumption and Risk of Cholecystectomy in Women." *American Journal of Medicine* 119:760–67.

Tseng, C. H., C. P. Tseng, C. K. Chong, T. P. Huang, Y. M. Song, C. W. Chou, S. M. Lai, T. Y. Tai, and J. C. Cheng. 2006. "Increasing Incidence of Diagnosed Type 2 Diabetes in Taiwan: Analysis of Data from a National Cohort." *Diabetologia* 49:1755–60.

Tsuda, Takanori, Yuki Ueno, Hitoshi Kojo, Toshikazu Yoshikawa, and Toshihiko Osawa. 2005. "Gene Expression Profile of Isolated Rat Adipocytes Treated with Anthocyanins." *Biochima and Biophysica Acta* 1733:137–47.

Turner, C. G. 1986. "What Is Lost with Skeletal Reburial? I. Adaptation." *Quarterly Review of Archaeology* 7:1–2.

Ubelaker, D. H., and L. G. Grant. 1989. "Human Skeletal Remains: Preservation or Reburial?" *Yearbook of Physical Anthropology* 32:249–87.

United States Government Documents. 1910. "Superintendent's Annual Narrative and Statistical Report from Field Jurisdiction, Cherokee Indian School." Microfilm 534, reel 1.

——. 1914. "Superintendent's Annual Narrative and Statistical Report from Field Jurisdiction, Cherokee Indian School." Microfilm 534, reel 1.

——. 1915. "Superintendent's Annual Narrative and Statistical Report from Field Jurisdiction, Cherokee Indian School." Microfilm 534, reel 1.

——. 1918. "Superintendent's Annual Narrative and Statistical Report from Field Jurisdiction, Cherokee Indian School." Microfilm 534, reel 1.

Urrutia-Rojas, Ximena, and John Menchaca. "Prevalence of Risk for Type 2 Diabetes in School Children." *Journal of School Health* 76(5):189–94.

van der Kolk, B. A., and R. E. Fisler. 1994. "Childhood Abuse and Neglect and Loss of Self-Regulation." *Bulletin of the Menninger Clinic* 58:145–68.

Vargas, Ileana. 2002. "Type 2 Diabetes in Children and Adolescents." http://abcnews.healthology.com/printer_friendlyAR.asp?f=diabetes&c=diabetes_type2 (accessed October 2002).

Van Doren, M., ed. *Travels of William Bartram.* New York: Dover, 1947.

Vitebsky, Piers. 1995. *The Shaman.* Boston: Little, Brown.

Wada, Leslie, and Boxin Ou. 2002. "Antioxidant Activity and Phenolic Content of Oregon Caneberries." *Journal of Agricultural and Food Chemistry* 50(12): 3495–3500.

Waldram, James B., D. Ann Herring, and T. Kue Young. 1995. *Aboriginal Health in Canada.* Toronto: University of Toronto Press.

Walker, P. L. 2000. "Bioarchaeological Ethics: A Historical Perspective on the Value of Human Remains." In *Biological Anthropology of the Human Skeleton,* ed. M. A. Katzenberg and S. R. Saunders, 3–39. New York: Wiley-Liss.

Wamala, S. P., J. Lynch, M. Horste, M. A. Mittleman, K. Schenck-Gustafsson, and K. Orth-Gomer. 1999. "Education and the Metabolic Syndrome in Women." *Diabetes Care* 22:1999–2003.

Wargovich, Michael J. 1999. "Experimental Evidence for Cancer Preventive Elements in Foods." *Cancer Letters* 114:11–17.

Waselkov, Gregory A. 1997. "Changing Strategies of Indian Field Location in

Early Historic Southeast." In *People, Plants, and Landscapes: Studies in Paleo-ethnobotany,* ed. K. J. Gremillion, 179–94. Tuscaloosa: University of Alabama Press.

Watkins, J. 1999. "Conflicting Codes: Professional, Ethical, and Legal Obligations in Archaeology." *Science and Engineering Ethics* 5:337–45.

Watkins, J., K. A. Pyburn, and P. Cressey. 2000. "Community Relations: What the Practicing Archaeologist Needs to Know to Work Effectively with Local and/or Descendant Communities." In *Teaching Archaeology in the Twenty-first Century,* ed. S. J. Bender and G. Smith, 73–81. Washington, DC: Society for American Archaeology.

Wehr, Demaris. 1987. *Jung & Feminism: Liberating Archetypes.* Boston: Beacon Press.

Weile, Marta. 1982. *Spiders and Spinsters: Women and Mythology.* Albuquerque: University of New Mexico Press.

Weiss, Kenneth M., Robert E. Ferrell, and Craig L. Hanis. 1984. "A New World Syndrome of Metabolic Diseases with a Genetic and Evolutionary Basis." *Yearbook of Physical Anthropology* 27:153–78.

Weiss, Kenneth M., R. E. Ferrell, C. L. Hanis, and P. N. Steyne. 1989. "Diabetes Mellitus in American Indians: Characteristics, Origins and Preventive Health Care." *Medical Anthropology* 11:283–304.

Weiss, Kenneth M., Jan S. Ulbrecht, Peter R. Cavanaugh, and Anne V. Buchanan. 1984. "Genetics and Epidemiology of Gallbladder Diseases in New World People." *American Journal of Human Genetics* 36:1259–78.

Welty, Thomas K. 1991. "Health Implications of Obesity in American Indians and Alaska Natives." *American Journal of Clinical Nutrition* 53(supp.):1616S–1620S.

Welty, Thomas K., and John L. Coulehan. 1993. "Cardiovascular Disease among American Indians and Alaska Natives." *Diabetes Care* 16(supp. 1):277–83.

Whitmont, Edward C. 1969. *The Symbolic Quest: Basic Concepts of Analytical Psychology.* Princeton: Princeton University Press.

Whittington, S. L. 1997. *Bones of the Maya: Studies of Ancient Skeletons.* Washington, DC: Smithsonian Institution Press.

*Who Owns the Past? The American Indian Struggle for Control of Their Ancestral Remains,* 2001, http://www.pbs.org/wotp/film_info/transcript/ (accessed August 2004 [site retired]).

Wiedman, Dennis William. 1989. "Adiposity or Longevity: Which Factor Accounts for the Increase in Type 2 Diabetes Mellitus When Populations Acculturate to an Industrial Technology?" *Medical Anthropology* 11:237–53.

Wilkins, Kathryn. 1996. "Tuberculosis, 1994." *Health Reports* 8(1):33–39.

Willey, G. R., and P. Phillips. 1958. *Method and Theory in American Archaeology.* Chicago: University of Chicago Press.

Willey, P. 1981. "Another View by One of the Crow Creek Researchers." *Early Man* 3:26.

Williams, Samuel Cole, ed. 1948. *Lieut. Henry Timberlake's Memoirs, 1756–1765.* Marietta, GA: Continental Book Company.

Willis, John T. 1984. "The First *Pericope* in the Book of Isaiah." *Vetus Testamentum* 34(1):63–77.

Winkelman, Michael. 1992. *Shamans, Priests and Witches: A Cross-Cultural Study of Magico-Religious Practitioners.* Anthropological Research Papers No. 44. Tempe: Arizona State University.

———. 2000. *Shamanism: The Neural Ecology of Consciousness and Healing.* Westport, CT: Gergin and Garvey.

Witthoft, John. 1946. "The Cherokee Green Corn Medicine and the Green Corn." *Journal of the Washington Academy of Sciences* 36(7):213–19.

———. 1949. "Green Corn Ceremonialism in the Eastern Woodlands." *Occasional Contributions from the Museum of Anthropology of the University of Michigan,* No. 13. Ann Arbor: University of Michigan Press.

———. 1977. "Cherokee Indian Use of Potherbs." *Journal of Cherokee Studies* 2(2):250–55.

———. 1983. "Cherokee Beliefs Concerning Death." *Journal of Cherokee Studies* 8(2):68–72.

———. n.d. *Cherokee Economic Botany.* Archives of the Philadelphia Historical Society.

Woloy, Eleanora M. 1990. *The Symbol of the Dog in the Human Psyche: A Study of the Human-Dog Bond.* Wilmette, IL: Chiron Publications.

Woodward, G. S. 1983. *The Cherokees.* Norman: University of Oklahoma Press.

World Archaeological Congress. 1989. "Vermillion Accord on Human Remains." South Dakota WAC Inter-Congress.

World Health Organization (WHO). 2002. "Statement by Dr Gro Harlem Brundtland Director-General of the World Health Organization on World Health Day, 7 April 2002." http://www.who.int/mediacentre/news/statements/statement03/en/index.html.

World Medical Organization. 1996. "Declaration of Helsinki." *British Medical Journal* 313:1448–49.

Wright, M. 1974. "A Metrical Analysis of the Morphological Relationship between Prehistoric Dallas and Historic Cherokee Skeletal Populations in East Tennessee." Master's thesis, University of Tennessee.

Wyatt, Sharon B., Karen P. Winters, and Patricia M. Dubbert. 2006. "Overweight and Obesity: Prevalence, Consequences, and Causes of a Growing Public Health Problem." *American Journal of the Medical Sciences* 331(4):166–74.

Yarnell, Richard A., and M. Jean Black. 1985. "Temporal Trends Indicated by a

Survey of Archaic and Woodland Plant Food Remains from Southeastern North America." *Southeastern Archaeology* 4(2):93–106.

Yeats, Karen, and Marcello Tonelli. 2006. "Indigenous Health: Update on the Impact of Diabetes and Chronic Kidney Disease." *Current Options in Nephrology and Hypertension* 15:588–92.

Youdim, K. A., B. Shukitt-Hale, S. MacKinnon, W. Kalt, and J. A. Joseph. 2000. "Polyphenolics Enhance Red Blood Cell Resistance to Oxidative Stress: In Vitro and in Vivo." *Biochima and Biophysica Acta* 1523:117–22.

Young, T. Kue. 1996. "Recent Health Trends in the Native American Population." In *Changing Numbers, Changing Needs: American Indian Demography and Public Health,* ed. G. D. Sandefur, R. R. Rindfuss, and B. Cohen. Washington, DC: National Academy Press.

Zennie, Thomas M., and C. Dwayne Ogzewalla. 1977. "Ascorbic Acid and Vitamin A Content of Edible Wild Plants in Ohio and Kentucky." *Economic Botany* 31:76–79.

Ziegler, Regina G. 1989. "A Review of Epidemiologic Evidence That Carotenoids Reduce the Risk of Cancer." *Journal of Nutrition* 119:116–22.

Zimmet, P. 2001. "Globalization, Coca-Colonization and the Chronic Disease Epidemic: Can the Doomsday Scenario Be Averted?" *Journal of Internal Medicine* February Supplement 741, 249(2):17–27.

# Contributors

**Heidi M. Altman** is an assistant professor of anthropology at Georgia Southern University. Her areas of study include Native American languages, language, culture, and identity, indigenous science systems, language shift, and language revitalization. She is currently working as a consultant with the Eastern Band of Cherokee Indians on language preservation and revitalization.

**Roseanna Belt** is an enrolled member of the Eastern Band of Cherokee Indians and director of the Western Carolina University Cherokee Center. She received her bachelor's degree in history from the University of Colorado–Boulder where she worked as a counselor for ten years. She earned her master's degree in counseling and consulting psychology from Harvard University's Graduate School of Education.

**Thomas N. Belt** is a native Cherokee speaker who was born in Tahlequah, NC. Tom is a Cherokee language coordinator and instructor at Western Carolina University (WCU). He attended the University of Oklahoma and the University of Colorado. He also assists the Culturally Based Native Health Program at WCU and helps coordinate language revitalization efforts in the Cherokee community.

**David N. Cozzo** received his bachelor's degree in biology from Eastern Kentucky University, his master's degree in Appalachian studies from Appalachian State University, and his Ph.D. in anthropology from the University of Georgia–Athens. His main areas of focus during his doctoral research were medical ethnobotany, nutritional ethnobotany, and human ecology of the southern Appalachian Mountains. He is currently the project director for the Revitalization of Traditional Cherokee Artisan Resources in Western Carolina University's Cherokee Studies Program.

**Michelle D. Hamilton** is a physical anthropologist and received her Ph.D. in anthropology from the University of Tennessee–Knoxville. She worked for the Eastern Band of Cherokee Indians as former Section 106 officer in the Tribal Historic Preservation Office (THPO) and consulted regarding NAGPRA and bioarchaeological issues for the tribe. Currently Michelle is an assistant professor of forensic anthropology at the University of Texas–San Marcos.

**Jenny James** is an independent research scholar with a background in comparative theology and religions. She received her Ph.D. in philosophical theology from the University of St. Michael's College, Toronto, in 1996. Her academic specialty is textual analysis. Currently she is preparing a monograph on the cultural history of the goddess and dog moiety in circumpolar religions from the Paleolithic period through the Iron Age.

**Susan Leading Fox** is an enrolled member of the Eastern Band of Cherokee Indians (EBCI). She earned her bachelor's degree from Warren Wilson College and her master's degree in social work from the University of North Carolina–Chapel Hill. She has worked for the EBCI health system and the Indian Health Service as a counselor and administrator. Currently Susan is the leading health official for the EBCI, the deputy health officer of the tribal Health and Medical Division. She oversees twenty-four health agencies for the tribe.

**Lisa J. Lefler** is the director of the Culturally Based Native Health Program and a visiting associate professor of anthropology at Western Carolina University (WCU). She is also a research associate at Wake Forest University's Department of Anthropology. Lisa received her Ph.D. in anthropology from the University of Tennessee–Knoxville in 1996. A medical and applied anthropologist with a focus in behavioral health, she has worked with the Eastern Band of Cherokee Indians as a behavioral science researcher focusing on diabetes prevention and youth, and has worked with the Indian Health Service regarding Native youth and addictions. She conducted research and taught at the University of Oklahoma and worked with their Indian Health Promotion Program. She is currently involved in the analysis of over three hundred interviews conducted among the Kiowa, Comanche, Apache, and Chickasaw nations of Oklahoma regarding American Indian fatherhood. She is a faculty member in WCU's Cherokee Studies Program and teaches health-related courses for the university's graduate certificate program in Native health.

**Russell G. Townsend** is the Tribal Historic Preservation Officer (THPO) and lead archaeologist for the Eastern Band of Cherokee Indians. He is an enrolled member of the Cherokee Nation of Oklahoma and is currently ABD in anthropology from the University of Tennessee–Knoxville.

# Index